FOUNDATIONS
OF
REIKI
RYŌHŌ

"Quite possibly the most comprehensive guide to the tradition of Reiki, Nicholas Pearson's *Foundations of Reiki Ryōhō* provides readers with everything they need to know in order to understand the first two levels of the Japanese healing art. Included is a detailed history of Reiki's origins as well as an impressive examination of the evolution of Reiki's sacred symbols. Pearson at once gives the reader a traditional understanding of the healing practice but also encourages the reader to explore, documenting some of the permutations of the tradition since its inception. I will be recommending this book to my own Reiki students."

STORM FAERYWOLF,
AUTHOR OF *AWAKENING THE BLUELOTUS:
A REIKI LEVEL ONE HANDBOOK* AND
BECOMING THE BLUELOTUS: A REIKI LEVEL TWO HANDBOOK

FOUNDATIONS OF

REIKI RYŌHŌ

A MANUAL OF
SHODEN AND OKUDEN

NICHOLAS PEARSON

Healing Arts Press
Rochester, Vermont • Toronto, Canada

Healing Arts Press
One Park Street
Rochester, Vermont 05767
www.HealingArtsPress.com

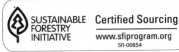

Text stock is SFI certified

Healing Arts Press is a division of Inner Traditions International

Note to the reader: *This book is intended as an informational guide. The remedies,
approaches, and techniques described herein are meant to supplement, and not to be a
substitute for, professional medical care or treatment. They should not be used to treat a
serious ailment without prior consultation with a qualified health care professional.*

Library of Congress Cataloging-in-Publication Data
Names: Pearson, Nicholas, 1986– author.
Title: Foundations of Reiki Ryōhō : a manual of shoden and okuden /
    Nicholas Pearson.
Description: Rochester, Vermont : Healing Arts Press, [2018] | Includes
    bibliographical references and index.
Identifiers: LCCN 2017029945 (print) | LCCN 2017031361 (e-book) |
    ISBN 9781620556733 (pbk.) | ISBN 9781620556740 (e-book)
Subjects: LCSH: Reiki (Healing system) | Spiritual healing.
Classification: LCC RZ403.R45 P43 2018 (print) | LCC RZ403.R45 (e-book) |
    DDC 615.8/52—dc23
LC record available at https://lccn.loc.gov/2017029945

Printed and bound in the United States by Lake Book Manufacturing, Inc.
The text stock is SFI certified. The Sustainable Forestry Initiative® program
promotes sustainable forest management.

10   9   8   7   6   5   4   3   2   1

Text design and layout by Virginia Scott Bowman
This book was typeset in Garamond Premier Pro with Morgan, Robato, and Cronos
Pro used as display typefaces
Illustrations by Steven Thomas Walsh unless otherwise noted

To send correspondence to the author of this book, mail a first-class letter to the
author c/o Inner Traditions • Bear & Company, One Park Street, Rochester, VT
05767, and we will forward the communication, or contact the author directly at
www.theluminouspearl.com.

CONTENTS

PART 1

Shoden: The First Degree

PART 2
Okuden: The Second Degree

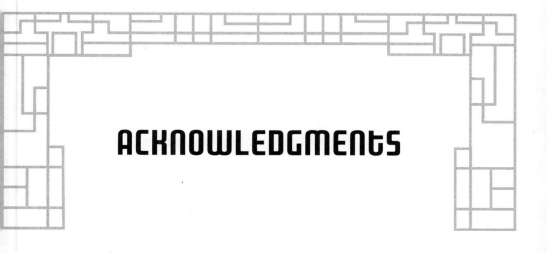

ACKNOWLEDGMENTS

THERE IS NO REIKI JOURNEY that does not include helpers, mentors, guides, and teachers. My personal journey to wholeness through Reiki is owed largely to my amazing teachers: Patricia Williams, Donna McMillan, Cindy Corry, and Frank Arjava Petter.

To Patricia: My deepest gratitude goes to you for first initiating me into the wonders of Reiki. Thank you for laying a firm foundation upon which my exploration could be built. I love you more than words can convey, and I am forever indebted to your kindness, compassion, and friendship. Most of all, thank you for living the Reiki Principles each day and inspiring me to do the same.

To Donna: Thank you for sharing the gift of *shinpiden* with me in Japan. Knowing you was a special gift, and I sincerely hope that your next journey on planet Earth is just as bright.

To Cindy: By teaching me Jikiden Reiki you broadened my horizons and helped me deepen my practice. Thank you for your continued support and friendship and for encouraging me to continue to grow with Reiki.

To Arjava: Your writing and research has inspired me for more than a decade now, and having the opportunity to study with you was a dream come true. Thank you for educating the Reiki community and continuing to dig deeper into the origins of the system of Usui Reiki Ryōhō. I appreciate you for sharing some additional stories about the history of Reiki with me; these vignettes nudged me in the right direction for some of the research in this book.

In addition to my wonderful Reiki instructors, I have overflowing gratitude for so many other wonderful Reiki friends and mentors. Richard Davis—I don't even know where to begin. Thank you for *all* of it. Our time together in Japan was an adventure I'll never forget, and visiting the birthplace of Reiki with you has forged memories that will last a lifetime. Thank you for your help in translating some of the Japanese in this book, as well as for helping me learn the language in the first place.

To Kathie Lipinski: Thank you for sharing your perspective and experience from your decades of teaching. I appreciate the time you took to share your insight with me and for offering feedback on the Reiki history chapter and the Japanese Reiki Techniques.

To Jojan Jonker: Thank you for your feedback on the manuscripts. I look forward to using it in future works.

To Audrey Pearson (no relation!): Thank you for consulting with Doi Hiroshi for historical data concerning the Usui Reiki Ryōhō Gakkai. Please send my regards to him and to the Gendai Reiki Hō Institute!

My dear Prudy Buehl is owed a mountain of thank-yous for helping to organize Reiki classes in her home. Together we have shared the Reiki teachings with a new generation of practitioners, and it is nothing but a delight to co-create with you. Your support has made all the difference in the world. Cheers to many more adventures together!

To my many more Reiki friends not yet named (I'm talking to you, Kat!): Thank you so much for encouraging me to write this book! Thank you to my students for being my test subjects as I wrote new curriculum and put together the manuscript. And thank you to my Reiki clients who came for treatments so I could ground myself firmly in Reiki as a practice, rather than being lost in its history or theory.

Most importantly: Thank you to my support system and artist extraordinaire—Steven Walsh. I appreciate everything you do and all that you are. I love you with all my heart. Thank you also to the wonderful team at Inner Traditions for helping transform the vision of this book into a reality. To my fabulous editor, Jamaica, I am especially grateful. You have once again helped shape my manuscript into a fully realized book, and for that I owe you an ocean of gratitude.

NOTES ABOUT ORTHOGRAPHY AND TERMINOLOGY

BECAUSE REIKI IS A JAPANESE PRACTICE, I have chosen to retain many of the original terms describing the history and use of Reiki. Japanese is written in a combination of complex characters and phonetic symbols, called *kanji* and *kana,* respectively. The Japanese terms are transcribed using the Hepburn romanization, a method that is more readable and pronounceable to speakers of English than most other methods. In most cases, the original Japanese characters are also provided for reference. Readers are encouraged to use the pronunciation guide and glossary of Japanese terms located in appendices B and C, respectively.

Except for proper nouns and words that have been adopted in English such as *kanji* and *sensei,* the Japanese words are italicized for ease in picking them out. Japanese naming conventions place the family name before a personal name, so that John Smith would be called Smith John in Japan. I have retained this convention throughout the text for individuals from Japan. In the case of the seminal Japanese-American Reiki teacher Hawayo Takata (1900–1980), I maintained Western conventions, with her personal name first and family name last. This is because she was a citizen born in Hawaii, which was at the time a territory of the United States. For convenience, a glossary of names important to the discussion of Reiki appears in appendix D.

Names in the glossary are alphabetized according to the style in which they appear in the text. Thus, Japanese names are listed with the family name first, while Western names are listed with personal name first.

The writing systems of the Japanese language have undergone revision and simplification throughout the last century. Wherever possible, the kanji that appear in this text reflect their forms from the era of Usui Mikao (1865–1926), the founder of Reiki Ryōhō. In other words, they are presimplified characters. Some of these older characters are no longer recognized by speakers of Japanese and they are becoming harder to translate. The glossary includes the modernized versions of many of these words to help readers and researchers undertake further study.

To the best of my knowledge, the transcriptions, translations, and original Japanese characters are as accurate as possible. Providing the original terms will hopefully facilitate further research despite the divide in history and culture between the birthplace of Reiki and the rest of the world.

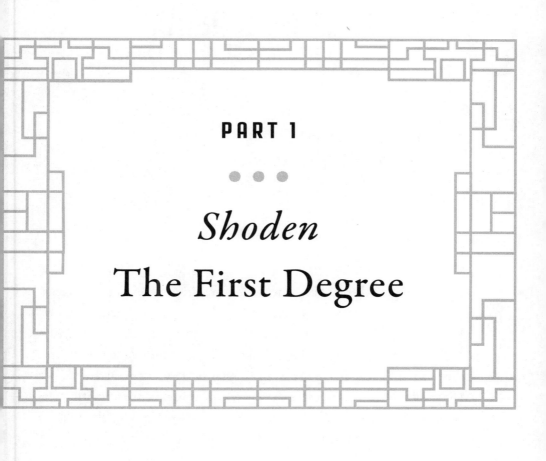

PART 1

• • •

Shoden

The First Degree

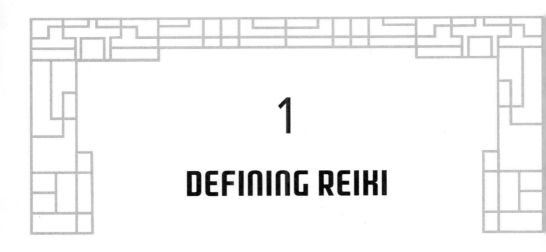

1

DEFINING REIKI

宇宙即我、即我宇宙

uchū ware soku, ware soku uchū

I am in the universe; the universe is in me

USUI MIKAO

REIKI IS KNOWN THE WORLD OVER as an effective system of relaxation, healing, and spiritual growth. The tradition of its practice stems from the efforts of Usui Mikao (1865–1926), a Japanese spiritual seeker who synthesized Reiki from his search for enlightenment in the early years of the twentieth century. Although the system of Reiki dates to its inception less than a century ago, it has undergone many leaps and changes along the course of its development. It is a simple and effective tool that anyone is capable of learning, and it offers tangible, practical results. The simplicity of Reiki is its appeal for most people who are brought to Reiki seminars, and for this reason it has proliferated worldwide.

In brief, Reiki Ryōhō is a healing art and spiritual tradition that grew out of Japanese culture. It is currently practiced as a hands-on healing modality in which practitioners become the conduit for the energy of Reiki to flow into themselves or another recipient. Reiki has been applied to a variety of physical, psychological, and spiritual conditions, with astonishing results. Today it is used by millions of people, including medical professionals and laypeople alike. The beauty of Reiki is that it is versatile, it requires no additional tools or equipment, and it can be learned by anyone who receives the initiation in a Reiki seminar. It has no contraindications, nor does it ever cause harm.

What we know as simply *Reiki* today is properly called Usui Reiki Ryōhō, meaning "Usui Reiki Healing Method." As mentioned above, Usui-sensei* (Usui Mikao) developed Reiki Ryōhō as a result of many years of study and practice in a number of different disciplines. A well-educated Japanese man who held a variety of professional posts throughout his life, he was first and foremost a spiritual seeker, which eventually led him to seek enlightenment by fasting on a mountaintop. When he had his awakening, or satori, in 1922 on Mount Kurama outside Kyoto, Japan, Reiki was born. Usui's desire was not to keep it secreted away as an obscure practice, nor did he want it to be owned wholly or in part by his family. Reiki's founder recognized that Reiki was so important and timely that it was for the entire world.

Nowadays, millions of Reiki practitioners represent hundreds of different forms or lineages of Reiki. Although all authentic systems can trace themselves back to Reiki's founder, Usui Mikao, the methodology and theory of systems can vary greatly from one to the next. My personal journey with Reiki has led me toward a more traditional approach. I enjoy the context of Reiki practice from a Japanese cultural and spiritual point of view. However, I treasure the fact that a Westernized lineage is what initially brought me to Reiki.

My teachers have been instrumental in helping me cultivate my daily practice. Reiki Ryōhō has changed my life, just as it has for countless other people across the planet. The blessings offered by this healing system are limitless; it may offer more than humankind will ever know.

Sensei is a suffix applied to someone's name to indicate respect. It usually means "teacher" and thus is used to indicate that the person so named may be an individual of high professional standing, or a teacher or instructor of some sort, such as *Takata-sensei* (Hawayo Takata) or *Chiyoko-sensei* (Yamaguchi Chiyoko). Anytime *Usui* or *Usui-sensei* is mentioned in the text as a stand-alone word or phrase, it refers to Usui Mikao.

Reiki is an intelligent force that needs no conscious direction to flow easily, without any command or effort on behalf of the practitioner. Reiki is almost too good to be true, especially because it is deceptively simple.

To really appreciate Reiki as an art form, it is necessary to look into what *Reiki* means. The traditionally accepted definition of *Reiki* among speakers of English is "universal life-force energy." The reason that the two short syllables that comprise the word are rendered as such a lengthy description is owed to the ideographic nature of the Japanese writing system. Words are depicted using characters borrowed from Chinese, which often convey several meanings, some of which are quite complex. Additionally, the cultural divide between Eastern and Western minds can require extra explanation.

REIKI ETYMOLOGY

Japanese orthography is comprised of several different character sets, including phonetic characters called *kana* and symbols called *kanji.* The written language of Japan was initially borrowed from that of the Han Chinese; in fact, *kanji* literally translates to "Han character." Over time, the written forms of these words evolved, resulting in differences between modern Chinese and Japanese characters. Furthermore, both languages underwent reformation to produce simpler characters as a means of making writing easier.

The origins of kanji are found in ancient pictographs carved into oracle bones. Many of these symbols were depictions of natural phenomena and daily experiences; they were graphic representations of the words. As the writing evolved, the characters themselves took on more stylized forms, and they would later convey more abstract ideas. By combining several basic symbols, called radicals, these abstract ideas could be better represented in written form.

Thus, kanji can be both pictographs (illustrations of objects and phenomena) and ideographs (abstract symbols conveying meaning). Some words can be produced from complex characters containing several radi-

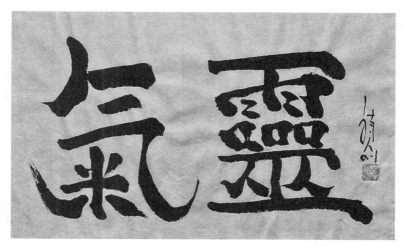

This illustration is of the word *Reiki* written in an older style of script. Note that the characters were originally written in reverse order (氣靈 instead of 靈氣) given that Japanese was once more commonly written right to left.
Calligraphy from the author's collection, photo by Steven Thomas Walsh

cals. Others, such as *Reiki,* are compound words comprised of multiple kanji. Compounds can be representations of an idea, such as 花火 (pronounced *hanabi*), for firework, whose characters translate individually as "flower" and "fire." This expression paints a mental picture of what a firework is. In other instances, new words in Japanese can be made of combinations of kanji and kana, resulting in many different parts of speech. Today there are over two thousand kanji in use in modern Japanese. They can be combined to produce countless new words.

Japanese characters typically have more than one pronunciation or reading, with most characters having at least two. In most cases, the different readings of a single character are grouped into the *on'yomi* and *kun'yomi.* The former is derived from the original pronunciation of characters in Chinese. Because the languages have different phonemes, the *on'yomi* are generally only approximations of how they initially sounded. *Kun'yomi* represent the native pronunciation of Japanese words.

Reiki was written as 靈氣 in Usui's time, though in today's simplified characters it is expressed as 霊気. It is a compound word, created from the joining of the words 靈 (rei) and 氣 (ki). The term *Reiki* in Japanese can be variously translated as "spirit energy," "aura," "soul energy," "ancestral energy," "miraculous energy," or "true self," among many other choices. *Reiki* was not an original word; Usui Mikao did not coin the term. Various methods and schools of healing with 靈氣 existed before Usui-sensei began to teach, although little historical information is available in English. *Reiki* is therefore a term that can have several layers of meaning, given that it is a product of the cultural, linguistic, and spiritual heritage of Japan.

Rei: 靈

The first symbol of *Reiki* is the *rei* component. It can be read as *rei, ryō, tama,* or *dama;* more obscurely, it is occasionally read as *hi, bi,* or *pi.* The symbol 靈 is often translated as "soul" or "spirit."* In Chinese, this character was variously used to mean "soul," "ghost," "elf," "bier," and "intelligence." As an adjective, it could describe something that was spiritual, universal, ancestral, intelligent, quick-witted, or effective.

The *rei* character is composed of several different radicals† that hint at its deeper meaning. The first radical is the symbol for rain, or *ame* (雨). This pictograph is meant to show raindrops falling from the sky. It can symbolize the blessings of the heavens raining down upon the earthly plane. Spiritual rain descends, reaching the crown of the skull, which is the same point where Reiki enters the practitioner. Rain is refreshing, cleansing, and rejuvenating, much like the practice of Reiki.

The second radical in the *rei* character is a series consisting of three square pictographs (example of pictograph: 口). This square pictograph

---

*Nowadays, this word has an uncomfortable connotation in modern Japanese. Though common in Usui's day, the *rei* character is seldom used except in words such as 幽霊 (yūrei) and 死霊 (shiryō), both of which mean "ghost." *Rei* is also used in several occult-related terms. For this reason, *Reiki* is frequently written in katakana as レイキ, the syllabary used for foreign loanwords as a means of circumventing the distaste or discomfort many Japanese individuals feel regarding this term.

†Radicals are the roots or component symbols within kanji. Some radicals represent the meaning of the word, while others are borrowed from similar-sounding words to indicate pronunciation. A character may be comprised of only a single radical, or it may contain many.

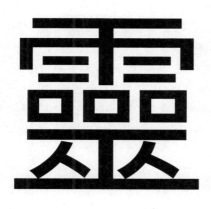 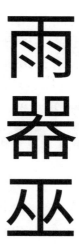

The character *rei* (left) is comprised of compressed or simplified versions of the radicals on the right.

usually means "mouth," but it can also indicate a vessel or bowl. In this case, the three boxes are a simplification of the kanji 器, pronounced *utsuwa,* which means "container" or "vessel." This part of the *rei* character teaches us to be the empty vessels for receiving the blessings of spiritual rain. Spiritual practitioners of all lineages must clear themselves, taking special care to set aside ego and attachment. The utsuwa radical helps us open, for if we are closed off or full of expectations, there is no room for the *ame* to enter and fill us.

Finally, the radical at the base of *rei* is 巫. It is originally the Chinese character for "shaman." In Japanese it is preserved in the word *miko* (巫女), which is a female attendant of a Shinto* shrine. Shinto is the endemic religion of Japan, the progeny of its native shamanism. Inside this character you can see the word for person repeated twice. This character, written as 人, is inside a larger framework that links the two people together. In similar fashion, the shaman is an intermediary, someone who acts as the link between the spiritual and material planes.

---

*Shinto (traditionally transliterated as *Shintō*) is the native religion of Japan. See chapter 3 for a discussion of Shinto.

The symbol for *rei* directs us to be the spiritual intermediaries of our time. As Reiki practitioners we release our judgments, attachments, and expectations so that we can be pure and open vessels for the spiritual blessings continuously bestowed by the universe. During the practice of laying on hands we become the conduit for Reiki energy to flow into the recipient. We serve as the link between the higher and lower realms so that Reiki can lead both practitioner and client toward balance.

Ki: 氣

The vital energy responsible for animating human beings and all living things is a concept shared by most cultures, ancient and modern. The word *ki* in Japanese, written as 氣, is identical to *chi* or *qi* in Chinese. This kanji is almost always pronounced *ki,* although it can sometimes be read as *ke.* It can mean "energy," "life force," "vitality," "spirit," "soul," or "mood." Similar terms in other languages include prana, mana, ruah, orgone, odic power, Wakan, telesma, and pneuma. Each of these indicates the vital power that animates life.

This kanji, like *rei,* is also a combination of radicals. The lower half is the pictograph of the rice plant: 米. Rice is a staple of the Chinese and Japanese diets. It is literally the fuel for the physical body, as it is the basis of the traditional meal. Since food is the source of metabolic energy, rice is metaphorically used to convey the spiritual energy that governs life. Ki is the sustenance of the soul, just as rice is nutrition for the body.

The upper radical in the *ki* character is 气, which is a pictograph for steam or vapor. It indicates something immaterial or intangible. Rather than merely being the literal fuel obtained from food, ki is instead the subtle or spiritual energy responsible for life. Ki or chi is considered to be the life force of every living thing. To the Eastern mind, ki isn't some inexplicable, mystical force; it is an everyday phenomenon that is part of the cultural paradigm. There are a wide number of expressions that use compound words containing the *ki* character, showing the prevalence of the idea in Japanese ideology.

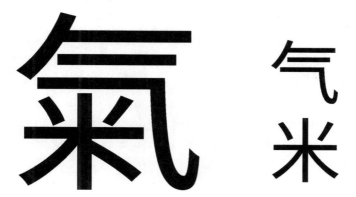

The character *ki* (left) is comprised of
the radicals on the right.

Some examples of ki-related terms include:

- 天気 (*tenki*): *weather,* literally "heaven ki"
- 気分 (*kibun*): *mood,* literally "ki minute," or "what you feel right now"
- 電気 (*denki*): *electricity,* literally "electric ki"
- 元気 (*genki*): *healthy,* literally "origin ki," or "health is the original state of being"
- 人気 (*ninki*): *popularity,* literally "person ki"
- 病気 (*byōki*): *illness* or *disease,* literally "sick ki"

All things have ki. Without it, there would be no movement or life in the universe. The various kinds of ki can be responsible for the function of blood, of breath, or even of thought. However, the most refined variety of ki in Japanese belief is Reiki. It is the divine or cosmic energy that brings our souls to life.

Reiki: 靈氣

If *rei* means "spiritual," "universal," "intelligent," and/or "effective," then 靈氣 or *Reiki* describes a spiritual form of ki that is spiritually or divinely guided. Reiki as an energy is universal because it is present in all beings, intelligent because it is from the most rarefied plane of existence, and effective because it can be used in the face of any illness, injury, or challenge. Reiki, the energy, is the driving force in Reiki Ryōhō, the healing system.

In the Japanese worldview, there are many categories of ki, each of which organizes or animates a different aspect of our makeup. There are seven main varieties that act directly upon our being and our experiences in life. Starting with the most basic and moving into the most rarefied, they are:

- *kekki* 血気, the ki of blood, which provides vitality
- *shioke* 塩気, the ki of salts or minerals, which offers structure
- *mizuke* 水気, the ki of water or liquids, which grants flux and communication
- *kuki* 空気, the ki of air, which grants breath
- *denki* 電気, the ki of thunder, which gives us motivation, striving, and growth
- *jiki* 磁気, the ki of magnetism, which endows us with complementary forces and challenges for growth
- *reiki* 霊気, the ki of soul, which is the same as 靈氣, the source of our healing system[1]

The final form of ki in this classification system is called *shinki* or 神気 (神氣 in presimplified kanji). This is the ki of the divine realm— the direct power of the creative principle of the universe. This is the energy from which we are all created and to which we return; however, it has no direct influence over material reality. Reiki, therefore, is the intermediary between our world of form and the plane in which *shinki* resides. It "is close enough to the principle of unity, as well as the principle of separation, to form an interface for the contact between the two . . . Reiki promotes all types of life process."[2]

Reiki is soul energy, or spirit energy. No person walking the face of the Earth is without a soul, so it stands to reason that we all share Reiki among the energies that are responsible for our lives. Reiki works principally at the soul level, meaning that it is spiritual healing rather than physical healing. Otherwise, we would call it "bodily guided life-force energy" or "materially guided healing." Since that isn't the case, we see that Usui-sensei was offering a system of healing that addressed all healing from the causal level of our existence: the soul itself.

Reiki is considered to be universal because it is equally available to all people for treating all conditions, without restriction or bias. It is applicable to everything by everyone. Reiki isn't just some part of the universe, it *is* the universe. Reiki moves in and through all things; Usui-sensei himself taught that all things have Reiki.[3] However, although Reiki as an energy is present in all things, being able to effectively use it in Usui Reiki Ryōhō requires an initiation, which awakens the practitioner to this aspect of his or her being.

Reiki is an intelligent force because it is divinely created and has no ego. During a treatment it reaches into the core of any situation without conscious direction or feedback from the practitioner. It just "knows" where to go because it recognizes our spiritual reality. Thanks to the intelligent, self-guided nature of Reiki energy, there is no contra-indication for its use. Reiki practitioners do not need to know the details of what is being treated, nor do they diagnose. The energy itself causes no harm, and it flows only through the practitioner to the recipient in a one-way stream. Thus, practitioners do not need protection, for there is no likelihood of taking on their client's energy or illness.

An alternate interpretation of the term 靈氣 is "true self."[4] Viewed from this vantage, Reiki is an intelligent force because it is the self behind the ego and persona; it wears no mask and can penetrate the veils we wear. Given that Reiki itself has no separation from the Divine (the "spiritual" aspect of the translation), it can remind us of our own innate connection.

Finally, Reiki is effective, or efficacious, because it reaches the level of our being where we are tied to the field of potentiality. If we heal at the physical level, then we are restricted by the laws of the material plane. This is why there are limitations to conventional medicine. However, when we heal at the level of the soul, anything is possible. Miracles can and often do take place when we practice Reiki. When we surrender our own egos and expectations, Reiki brings balance.

A natural homeostatic mechanism exists in the human body and is also found in the immaterial levels of our makeup. It is self-correcting and self-equilibrating. Reiki supports these efforts by catalyzing change and eliminating the toxins or attachments that stand in the way of our well-being. The most commonly discussed benefit of Reiki is stress reduction; naturally, when we feel less stress we experience healing of the body, mind, and spirit. However, Reiki's healing influence is much deeper than that which is provided by the relaxation it offers. Reiki taps into our divine potential to live, love, and create unimaginable joy and success.

I'm often asked to define what Reiki is, and like many other practitioners and teachers, I often find myself without a clear and simple answer. Reiki encompasses so much more than words can articulate, so I don't have a rote response when asked by Reiki newcomers to describe what this energy really is. My first teacher put it best, though, and I often find myself returning to her words: "Reiki is unconditional love."

In my own experience, love is a concept that both practitioners and laypeople can relate to easily. Love is the creative principle and organizing force of the universe; unconditional love is at the core of all spiritual traditions. When we think of Reiki as love, it isn't just the motherly love and tenderness of caring for someone who is ill, though it is that, too, sometimes. Love is a cosmic energy that resides in every particle and wave of Creation. It's the true nature from which we are created and to which we aspire. Love is perfect balance, and Reiki is a mechanism of that love within our beings, which are seeking a return to wholeness.

Usui Reiki Ryōhō: Reiki as a Healing Art

When Usui Mikao developed the system of Reiki in the first half of the twentieth century, he called it 心身改善臼井靈氣癒法 or Shin Shin Kaizen Usui Reiki Ryōhō, which means "Usui Reiki Healing Method for Improving the Heart-Mind and Body." He was stressing the importance that healing first takes place in the mind, which is written with the pictograph for heart in Japanese: 心 (usually read as *kokoro* or *shin*).

Reiki as a healing art cultivates a relationship with Reiki the energy as a means of bringing the mind back into balance. Essentially, the outcome of diligent Reiki practice is no different than the mental and spiritual training found in most of the world's religions.

The paradigm that dominates in most branches of Reiki practice is that it is a spiritual art that aims to deliver physical, mental, and emotional healing. However, evidence provided by researching the original Reiki teachings of Usui Mikao tells us otherwise. When he gave birth to Reiki Ryōhō, Usui wasn't seeking a means of healing; his goal was attainment of inner peace. Indeed, Usui's initial teachings focused on Reiki Ryōhō as a spiritual path. Healing was a natural, though secondary, benefit of the spiritual work.

Usui Reiki Ryōhō began through a series of interdisciplinary spiritual studies enacted by Usui Mikao. He described its origin thusly: "I have not been taught this art of healing by anyone under the heavens, nor have I studied in order to obtain this mysterious ability to heal. I accidentally realized that I was given this mysterious healing ability when I felt the great power and was inspired by the mystery during a period of fasting."[5] As we will explore later, he was a seeker for much of his life, and he applied his natural curiosity and spiritual hunger to many different religions and traditions. He received Reiki through an ascetic practice on top of Mount Kurama. According to the memorial stone erected by his students following Usui's death in 1926, after weeks of fasting he "felt a great Reiki over his head."[6]

This "great Reiki" or 大靈氣 (pronounced *dai Reiki*) was the energy Usui-sensei felt when his awareness opened to the spiritual truth of his existence. Usui felt a deep sense of communion with Source, or Creator, and his mind naturally found deep peace. In this state Usui experienced true oneness or nonduality. The resultant state of inner peace is called 安心立命 or *anshin ritsumei* in Japanese. It is imperturbable and marks spiritual enlightenment, or satori. It is in this state that one is most able to accomplish the divine purpose of one's life.

When Usui Mikao realized the potential of Reiki for improving the mind and the body, he developed ways to transmit his experience of *anshin ritsumei.* Usui is known to have taught thousands of students in his lifetime, and it is likely that he adapted his teachings to meet the skill set and developmental level of the individuals drawn to his teachings. For some people, Reiki would have been simply a healing method; for others it would prove to be a path to enlightenment.

HOW REIKI IS PRACTICED TODAY

Reiki as a system has grown and evolved since its inception as a formal practice in the 1920s. Since that time, this healing tradition has spread across the globe and touched the lives of millions of people. Although Reiki has changed forms and has occasionally been imbued with add-ons by the generations of teachers who have succeeded Usui Mikao, all genuine Reiki lineages share the following attributes:

- Initiation
- The five precepts
- Treatment
- Progressive degrees
- Symbols (and mantras)
- Personal development

These six elements of Reiki serve as the common DNA in each of the branches in Reiki's family tree. Although various Reiki systems have different outer forms that these elements take—such as a unique initiation or attunement ritual for each lineage—all forms of Reiki must incorporate these six qualities or components. Traditional Reiki, both Eastern and Western, serves as the foundation for how these elements have manifested in each Reiki lineage worldwide.

Initiation

One aspect of Reiki that sets it apart from other energy-based healing modalities is that it is an initiatory system. The form and number of initiations vary between lineages. Despite this variance, each method works. Japanese forms of Reiki practice call this initiatory experience *reiju* (靈授).

Initiation confers healing ability through communion with the universal Reiki that lies in each of us. The act of initiation is sometimes called an "attunement," because it is believed to adjust the student's energy system in order for him or her to connect with Reiki as a healing force. And initiation is a permanent process; once established, the connection to Reiki is immediate and lasting. Lack of practice does not cause your ability to channel Reiki to atrophy. However, regular practice does strengthen your channel.

Initiation or attunement works by clearing away the mental, emotional, and spiritual debris that inhibits experience of your true nature. Your identity is not related to the material world; it isn't your body, your career, your name. The real you *is* Reiki. There is no separation between you and the spiritually guided energy that radiates from Source. The initiation serves as your *initial* experience of the ultimate truth. Because of this, many people experience a detoxifying reaction to the attunement itself because they are coming back into balance after having been out of touch with their spiritual identity.

I like to think that the most beautiful and mysterious aspect of Reiki is the initiation itself. Many people experience strong sensations, emotions, or other events before, during, and after the ceremony. Whether you receive only one attunement in your life or participate in monthly meetings that include initiation, it never ceases to be a spiritual experience. There is some mystical part of Reiki that guides the actual essence of the attunement, so that after the physical actions are completed, the student is forever changed for the better.

Finally, initiation into Reiki also confers your lineage. You cannot be attuned to Usui Reiki Ryōhō if it cannot be traced back to Usui Mikao. All authentic Reiki systems can map their family tree back to Usui-sensei, and it is vital to confirm this lineage before enrolling in a Reiki seminar. The importance of lineage isn't to tell you who is better pedigreed or who has influenced whom, for these concepts appeal to the ego rather than the heart (*kokoro*). Unless we all prepare ourselves for death on a mountaintop, we cannot expect to have the awakening experienced by the founder of Reiki Ryōhō. Therefore, we rely upon someone who has had the Reiki activated in them, thus conferring the ability to practice Reiki—and to teach it in kind to us.

You cannot give what you don't have; it's just that simple. Reiki initiations are performed *in person* for the same reason. Although there may be some spiritual dedicants out there who are at the necessary level of evolution to confer *reiju* over a distance, they are few and far between. Similarly, the recipient would have to be equally as prepared to *receive* this gift in the same way. There is an important bond between teacher and student, and Reiki incorporates this through both instruction and initiation.

Many words are now used for this element of the Reiki system: *reiju, attunement, empowerment, initiation, transmission of light,* and *transformation* each describe the experience. This part of Reiki practice should be treated reverently; handing out attunements en masse without any respect helps neither the recipients nor Reiki itself. Take time to compartmentalize the *reiju* in one way or another so that its sanctity is emphasized by setting it apart from the rest of a Reiki seminar.

As a prospective student, you can prepare yourself for your initiation by eating in a healthier manner, cutting back on stimulants and alcohol, reducing meat intake, and spending more time in nature. Meditation, exercise, yoga, and other practices can prepare your heartmind as well as your body for the sacred experience of a Reiki attunement. Be gentle with yourself and reduce your exposure to the media and the relentless stream of bad news it delivers so that you stay centered and nurture your spiritual heart. Each of these activities can enhance your attunement.

The Five Principles

When Usui Mikao formalized his system in order to impart it to others, he summarized his teachings in the *gokai* (五戒), which means "five admonitions" in Japanese. These few short statements are articulated in one of the few surviving documents that can accurately be attributed to Usui himself. The *gokai* became the Reiki Principles or Reiki Ideals when the first Western students were taught.

This initial teaching of Western students was done by Hawayo Takata, who was a very important figure in Reiki's history. Born in Hawaii in 1900, she was a Japanese-American Reiki practitioner who helped bring the Japanese healing art to the West through her teachings and promotion of it.

The Five Principles are the spiritual backbone of the Usui System, and they continue to be as relevant to the people of today as they were in 1920s Japan. The Reiki Principles will be described in detail in a later chapter, but in short they can be stated as:

> Just for today:
> Do not anger.
> Do not worry.
> Be grateful.
> Be diligent in your work.
> Be kind to others.

The rendering of these statements in English (and other languages) varies greatly from source to source, although the spirit of the ideals remains. These five simple directives, as well as their preface of "just for today," serve as spiritual, moral, and ethical guidelines for practitioners of Reiki at all levels.

It can be argued that Reiki, in its genesis, was primarily a *spiritual* practice, rather than one related to health and healing, so the Five Principles or *gokai* were introduced to help students navigate along their journey. Usui taught that all illness first occurs in the mind or spirit (*kokoro*), and thus the *gokai* are tools for achieving healing at the core level. When we practice them, we become happier, healthier, more successful individuals. Healing is a natural result of bringing the mind back into balance.

Usui originally guided his students to practice these precepts daily; the entire text of the *gokai* as he wrote it included instructions for reciting the principles morning and evening, as well as keeping them in the heart. Many Reiki lineages today do not offer more than a cursory glance at the Reiki Principles, and a few lineages omit them entirely. Even those whose primary focus is on physical healing often relay the *gokai* in one form or another as part of the first degree (*shoden*) teachings.

In order to maintain Usui's legacy and maintain the integrity of the Reiki system, the principles need to be practiced. What separates Usui Reiki Ryōhō from other forms of healing (including other forms of Reiki in Japan) is the fact that it is Usui's method. These short statements may seem simple, but they are deceptive in their depth and breadth. We learn mindfulness, compassion, devotion, and presence when we actively use the *gokai*. Everything else in the system of Reiki as it was originally taught is secondary to these teachings. We will examine their origin and meaning in depth at a later point.

Treatment

For most people, the aspect of treating themselves or their loved ones is the motivating force behind learning Reiki. Although the form that treatment takes can differ wildly from one lineage to the next—not unlike the many varieties of initiation—all of them work, which is one of the mysteries of Reiki. Treatments can be performed on oneself or on another individual; they can be local treatments or they can be remote. Reiki works its wonders in restoring balance in any case.

The foundation of most Reiki traditions is treatment. In virtually any first degree class, the instructor will emphasize the importance of treatment. Self-treatment is prescribed to counteract the twenty-one-day cleansing or integration period following the initiation. Self-treatment is also recommended as the best way to grow your budding Reiki skills. The more we use it on ourselves, the more sensitive we become to the energetic aspect of healing and the more proficient we are at responding to that energy. Hayashi Chūjirō, one of Usui's *shihan* or teachers whom we will discuss more later, described the system as very practical. An article from the *Hawaii Hochi* reports Hayashi's description of Reiki as follows: "Reiki Ryōhō is not a psycho-spiritual therapy, it is not prayer therapy, it is not a charm or incantation, it is not so-called quackery, but it is an exceedingly **rational** therapy."[7]

Despite the outer differences in the many methods of applying Reiki, the mechanism at work never changes. There is no complicated ritual necessary, nor is any mental trigger required. Hawayo Takata and Jikiden Reiki founder Yamaguchi Chiyoko, both direct students of Hayashi-sensei, used to instruct, "Hands on, Reiki on; hands off, Reiki off!" Reiki treatment works wherever you are, and it needs no preamble or prop. It flows as it is needed.

Reiki can be practiced discreetly in public, with a palm placed against a thigh or on the stomach. It can be offered to a loved one during an embrace. Reiki can be shared anytime, anywhere; use it while you attend a concert or visit the movie theater. Use it at the dinner table and as you drift off to dreamland. Reiki is versatile and nurturing, so you can adapt it to your needs. Although it is easy to place a hand on yourself or a loved one while you are engaged in another activity, the best results are always gleaned when you set aside time for Reiki.

It is used to treat a wide variety of conditions. Starting with the easiest, Reiki is safe and effective for stress, anxiety, depression, fatigue, and much more. My own experience with Reiki for pain management has bordered on the miraculous. I have seen it treat burns in a matter of minutes, heal open wounds in days and sometimes hours, expedite the knitting together of broken bones, and overcome the common cold. Reiki knows no limits.

Many individuals who are drawn to Reiki are looking to benefit in the face of chronic and terminal conditions. Reiki has been used in palliative and rehabilitative scenarios with great success. Scientific and medical literature is beginning to document the effects of Reiki treatment in cases of cancer, dementia, and many more conditions. In situations such as these, regular treatment every day is the key to seeing results.

Reiki treatment is based upon the tradition of *tenohira* and *teate* in Japan. These are hands-on healing practices, meaning literally "palm healing" and "hand placement." A long tradition of *tenohira* is evident among Japanese spiritual movements; Reiki is only one of many. Laying on of hands has been used among many cultures as a means of effecting change in an individual's health. Sects of Christianity continue to use it today, as do many other types of healers.

Touch, by its very nature, is therapeutic. In a world of disconnection, making conscious and conscientious contact with another person can offer something that is otherwise entirely absent from the lives of some people. To touch without agenda or motive—merely being present and mindful—is one of the greatest gifts of Reiki. The added bonus is that the flow of Reiki energy enhances, supports, and supercharges that loving, compassionate contact.

Reiki is administered today with gentle touch; there is no need to press or manipulate for Reiki to flow. Similarly, the mind is not required to direct or focus Reiki in any specific manner. Practitioners are simply the empty vessels through which the universal energy is poured. Still your mind and connect to Reiki in whatever manner is meaningful to you; Reiki will respond.

We know today that Usui himself often used a combination of techniques for healing. After the Great Kanto Earthquake of 1923 it is said that he would treat up to six people at once: one with each hand and each foot, one with his eyes, and one with his breath. Usui-sensei also instructed his students to pat, rub, and tap Reiki into clients, as well as to "beam" it by using a special mudra-like hand position. Today, Reiki is usually practiced more simply, especially by beginners.

Treatment can be performed in a hands-off method, too. This is especially helpful when legislation does not permit practitioners to make physical contact without proper licensure or training (such as exists in massage therapy or nursing license). Hands-off healing is conducted with the hands just above the body of the recipient. When some people are uncomfortable with practitioner-to-client contact, the hands-off method is acceptable. In first aid scenarios, physical touch may be too painful, such as in the case of cuts, burns, scrapes, and other injuries; in these cases Reiki can be given hands-off and/or with the eyes and breath.

In the higher degrees of Reiki training, practitioners also learn to use Reiki remotely. Long-distance healing has a long-standing precedent for success, and Reiki is no exception. Without the *okuden* initiation and training, however, practitioners are not equipped with the tools needed to connect as deeply. Newcomers to the Reiki system often do report success, however, by intending that Reiki flow to a nonlocal target.

Many lineages prescribe a specific treatment protocol using designated hand placements. The same positions are used in every complete treatment. Others prefer a more intuitive approach wherein Reiki practitioners are encouraged to place their hands wherever they are led to do so. Both methods have value; whichever works for you will do the job. Personally, I have found that a foundation practice of hand placements works like having training wheels on your bike. Treating the entire person ensures that Reiki will go where it's most needed. As you practice more and more, you learn to listen to your guidance, and your hands are sensitized to where Reiki will have the greatest impact.

To reiterate an important point, no matter the form of treatment, Reiki can never do harm. Reiki is an intelligent force that knows where to treat and how much to offer. There is no such thing as too much Reiki, or a case where Reiki can make a condition worse. In some instances, recipients experience a "healing reaction" or "healing crisis" wherein symptoms intensify initially. This happens as the body, mind, and spirit address the underlying issue of disease; with continued treatment the healing reaction lessens, and the condition generally disappears in time, too.

Progressive Degrees

In the majority of lineages, Reiki training is offered in three progressive levels. Unique tools and techniques are offered at each level, with the overall focus deepening as your training progresses. The three degrees of Western Reiki are a perfect adaptation of the three levels of Japanese-style Reiki; Usui-sensei taught them by the names of *shoden, okuden,* and *shinpiden.* Each of the three levels was generally broken down into smaller, more manageable sections.

Students of Reiki must begin with the first degree, or *shoden,* class. The initial seminar offers the very first initiation to fledgling practitioners so that they may open to the experience of channeling Reiki energy. Following this, some teachers will require a waiting period before offering level two, though many present both classes together. Usui-sensei preferred that students developed their sensitivity before he permitted them to proceed with their training at the *okuden* level. The remainder of Reiki training consists of the third degree, which prepares practitioners to become teachers.

Although there are teachers who provide accelerated classes, such as initiating students as Reiki Masters by teaching all three degrees in a single weekend, this method is generally frowned upon. When practitioners have time to assimilate the information and apply the treatments, meditations, symbols, and precepts, they will be more effective later on. There is no substitute for practice, so most Reiki teachers will encourage students to master the basics in each degree before moving on.

Different lineages and styles of Reiki may have a different number of levels available (and we know that Usui's original format differs from most of those offered today). The different levels available are a result of the three degrees either having been broken into smaller sections or having been given additional material. Generally speaking, more levels do not necessarily make a better system. Since all varieties of Usui Reiki Ryōhō originate from the same source and the same energy, following our first initiation we all have the same Reiki-infused hands and hearts.

Be sure to find the style that best suits you and progress as you are driven to do so.

Symbols

At higher degrees of initiation, practitioners are taught several symbols that enhance the goals of Reiki. In most cases, three traditional symbols are taught at level two and one at level three. There is a fair amount of deviation in this, as some lineages provide the first symbol with the first degree class, whereas others have added to the number of symbols in their teachings. Even more confusing, there is evidence that the fourth symbol, often referred to as the master symbol, may have been added to Usui Shiki Ryōhō, which is Reiki as traditionally taught by Hawayo Takata. Although the symbols themselves are not provided in this text, we can look broadly at the function and origin of Reiki symbols as a whole. (Additionally, an in-depth discussion of each of the *okuden* symbols is provided in part 2.)

If we were to travel back in time to when Usui Mikao first began teaching others from his perspective of *anshin ritsumei,* we would probably witness something that shares very little with today's Reiki Ryōhō of any variety. If you recall, *reiju* initially consisted of simply sharing space in total silence with Usui-sensei. Perhaps the student stared into the teacher's eyes in contemplative focus as the latter helped awaken the pupil to the experience of the *dai Reiki* that awakened him. The harsh reality of this scenario is that few students were truly able to access Reiki through this experience, as it required that a rigorous, disciplined spiritual practice be in place beforehand.

We know from Usui-sensei's memorial stone and from an interview with him preserved in the handbook* issued by the Usui Reiki Ryōhō Gakkai (Usui's Reiki Healing Society, founded by Usui himself) that the founder did not want to keep Reiki under wraps. He wanted this system of self-actualization and healing to span the globe. In order to make this a reality, he adapted his system and added tools that were more appropriate for laypeople. Among these number the formalized meditations, ritualized *reiju,* teachings about *byōsen* and healing, and the introduction of the symbols to Reiki.

The symbols themselves fall into classes of pure symbols, often called *shirushi* in Japanese, and *jumon.* The former class is drawn from ancient traditions, whereas *jumon* are formulations derived from modern kanji. The names of the symbols found in Westernized branches of Reiki act like mantras and can be used on their own to the same ends as the

---

*This handbook is called *Usui Reiki Ryōhō Hikkei,* and it is still used by the *gakkai* today. The *gakkai* has an additional booklet called *Reiki Ryōhō no Shiori* that was published in 1974.

symbols. The Reiki symbols can be used as adjuncts to the healing process and applied to many situations in life. (More detailed information will be provided in the *okuden* manual in part 2 of this book.)

The symbols are tools; they are not required to practice Reiki. However, they can augment and transform your practice. Use them with respect; they are powerful spiritual catalysts. With regular practice, we actually embody what the symbols represent. In this way the symbols are like training wheels; they are meant to help us until we can work beyond them.

Personal Development

Although most practitioners are drawn to Reiki as a healing modality, every person that I have known to learn Reiki Ryōhō experiences transformation on one level or another. Wherever seeds of Reiki are planted, they seem to blossom into more than simple wellness. Reiki Ryōhō is something greater than most of us can conceive; it is a direct connection to Source. Usui-sensei summed up this in the enigmatic expression *uchū ware soku, ware soku uchū* (宇宙即我、即我宇宙). Though a literal translation is not possible, it roughly means "I am in the universe, and the universe is in me."

Reiki empowers you to take your life into your own hands. Just knowing that you can create change by laying your hands on a problem area in your body is enough to affect most people's psyche. Witnessing Reiki miracles and serving others with your Reiki hands is profound; there is nothing else like it that I've experienced. Even the staunchest, most skeptical of individuals may begin to have a spiritual experience during a Reiki treatment. This is one of Reiki's many gifts.

Personal development can manifest as better and healthier life decisions or even just a change in attitude. More than likely, though, practitioners who practice regularly will see a vast improvement in their inner and outer worlds. Reiki permeates all that you do in order to bring greater balance of body, mind, and spirit. Reiki offers an abundance of blessings in order to awaken your consciousness to a higher reality.

Usui-sensei clearly wanted Reiki to help others accomplish their purpose in life. Some sources claim that prior to the formalization of Usui Mikao's teachings, his students merely knew his teachings as "Usui's way" or "Usui's method for self-actualization." The founder of Reiki was developing a system for reaching our highest potential; the *gokai,* hands-on healing, initiation, symbols, and other tools offered at each degree are merely stepping-stones on the path to self-realization.

Some scholars and practitioners posit that the Usui System is primarily aimed at healing, whereas others want to peel back the veil of wellness and see more deeply into Reiki. On the surface, we might be opening to the laying on of hands for better health. However, I believe that these external changes we experience are actually underscoring the true goal of Reiki: enlightenment, or *anshin ritsumei.*

For all who are called to it, Reiki is available to help us achieve our own spiritual awakening. To do so often requires addressing the most pressing needs first, such as a broken bone or asthma. As we bring our bodies and minds back into greater balance with the tools that Reiki grants to us, we are removing all the barriers on the path to authentic liberation and awakening.

❖ Reiki Reflections: Your Own Definition

After reading about the background of Reiki and discovering how it works on several different levels, you're likely to have formed a clear picture of what Reiki means. Take some time to write out your own definition of Reiki in a manner that is meaningful to you. Compare it to the descriptions of your classmates if you are enrolled in a Reiki seminar or ask friends who are also practitioners. Notice how each person likely tailors their depiction of Reiki according to his or her personal experience.

When you map out your personal definition of Reiki, try to select a translation of the Reiki kanji that feels comfortable to you and supports your understanding of what Reiki is, both as an energetic force and as a healing system. After your initiation, has that definition changed? Revisit this definition after a month, six months, or even a year after your first initiation. How much has your conception and understanding of Reiki been shaped by your practice?

2

LEARNING REIKI

MORE THAN ONE of the six major elements of Reiki relate to how the system is taught. Reiki is special among healing practices because of its initiation ceremony that confers the ability on new practitioners. Because of this unique aspect of Reiki, no extended training or cultivation is required in order to apply it in practical situations. Initiations also delineate the separate levels of the Reiki system. Traditionally, Western branches of Reiki utilize three degrees, sometimes broken up into more than one class each. Eastern forms of Reiki laid the framework with this, as they have three overarching degrees of Reiki training.

With every opportunity to receive initiation, practitioners experience a refinement in their inner vessel; their ability to channel Reiki expands and improves. Although the initiation generally has a permanent effect, successive *reiju* or initiations enhance the process begun in your level one class. For this reason, many lineages offer more than one initiation in the *shoden* class, and practitioners are encouraged to continue their studies with Reiki in the successive degrees.

Below we will take a look at the various levels of Reiki according to how they are most often taught. Initiations are a sacred ceremony, so the exact details will not be discussed in this book; they also differ greatly in outer form from one branch of Reiki to another. Bear in mind that some teachers make changes of their own accord, and some styles of Reiki differ from the norm as well. When preparing for your own Reiki classes, you should be encouraged to find out exactly what each degree entails.

THE INITIATION

In Japanese, the initiation is called *reiju,* written as 靈授 in kanji. The first character should look very familiar; it is the same *rei* in *Reiki.* The second symbol means "to grant," "to offer," or "to teach." *Reiju* is a spiritual offering; it confers or grants the ability to become the empty vessel through which the great Reiki of the universe pours itself. *Reiju* is a spiritual gift that awakens you to your authentic self, which is never separate from Reiki, for Reiki is the spiritual ki resident in all things.

Reiju is not an isolated concept; it is used in tandem with the expression 靈受, also pronounced *reiju.* In this instance, the second *reiju* means "to receive soul/spirit." When an initiation is performed, the Reiki Master/Teacher offers a spiritual gift and the student receives said gift. Initiation is not received with the mind or the body; it is given soul to soul and must therefore be received on the spiritual plane. We know that Usui-sensei initially had no formal ritual for initiating new individuals into Reiki Ryōhō; he merely held the space for them to receive the *reiju* at the soul level. Since most practitioners today are not at the level that Usui Mikao was, we use physical rituals to enhance the process of giving and receiving initiations.

Usui maintained that students would benefit from receiving frequent *reiju.* In Japan, traditional lineages of Reiki—including the Usui Reiki Ryōhō Gakkai, founded by Usui-sensei himself—participate in monthly *reijukai,* or "initiation meetings." Repeated initiation helps to refine one's ability to serve as a conduit for Reiki and improve one's ability as a practitioner. Furthermore, since the *reiju* itself was meant as a substitute for Usui-sensei's austere meditation on Mount Kurama, *reiju* is also a tool for spiritual awakening, or satori. Practitioners of all lineages often report similar experiences during and after an initiation; they resemble the first steps toward attaining *anshin ritsumei.*

Many Western Reiki teachers describe a twenty-one-day integration period that takes place after each attunement. Students are warned that they may experience any number of symptoms as their bodies react to Reiki energy. These conditions may include dizziness, digestive distress, fever, pain, fatigue, feeling energized, better or worse sleep, more vivid dreams, enhanced psychic perception, reduced pain, and much more. The idea is that we are all unique, and therefore we will respond to the initial awakening of Reiki energy within us differently. There is no set period for integrating this, but twenty-one days is a good estimate. Although this twenty-one-day cycle is a product of Western thinking,* it is experienced by many new practitioners as they open to the energy of Reiki.

While ostensibly it may appear that the goal of the initiation, or *reiju,* is to confer the ability to practice Reiki, this is merely the by-product of the ceremony. If we shift our thinking away from the paradigm of an "attunement" to Reiki, we can view *reiju* as the initiation into a higher state of consciousness. This expanded awareness isn't necessarily mystical. The initiation is simply a spiritual tool to provoke you into having an *initial* experience of your true nature.

The Reiki initiation is sometimes called an *empowerment, transformation,* or *transmission.* In fact, early writings on Reiki Ryōhō dating to the late 1920s refer to the type of instruction as *denju* in Japanese.[1] Written originally as 傳授, and now as 伝授 in simplified kanji, this term indicates that a spiritual offering or empowerment is passed on or transmitted from teacher (the Reiki Master or *shihan*) to student, to aid in the student's development. The term *denju* has fallen out of use in modern Reiki Ryōhō, although it is still commonly used in Buddhism and other Japanese spiritual sects to describe the act of initiation or empowerment.

Reiki is inherently spiritual. Although many professional practitio-

---

*The likeliest origin of the twenty-one-day cycle of cleansing and integration stems from the commonly held belief that a new habit requires twenty-one days to take hold. If new Reiki practitioners expect that they will have the above symptoms, they are much more likely to want to give themselves Reiki every day during that period. Thus, the habit of self-care is built into the practice from the beginning of one's Reiki journey.

ners and teachers have sanitized their teachings of the more esoteric or foreign elements to make them seem mainstream, thereby helping to establish Reiki programs in hospitals, shelters, and other facilities, the mystery of Reiki still lingers at the heart of the system. And without the sacred experience of initiation, it is not possible to become a Reiki practitioner.

Many talented healers are hard at work providing the world with viable tools; they do not all use Reiki, however. The Reiki initiation instantly connects new students to the universal flow of Ki by offering a clear glimpse into their own limitless nature. This is why Reiki is such an effective method of healing, and one that never depletes the practitioner. The empowerment itself provides a permanent connection to an ever-flowing stream of Reiki energy.

As touched upon earlier, the way that initiations or attunements are performed is sometimes wildly different among the many branches of Reiki. Some factions have no discernible ritual, while others include precise sequences of symbols and breathing. Some later additions to the Reiki family tree have incorporated aspects from qigong and some New Age practices into their attunements, whereas others have chosen to simplify. Some teachers even claim to send attunements remotely, as well as via books, DVDs, and Internet videos. In spite of documents proving that Takata-sensei performed remote initiations in rare circumstances,* we have no indication as to how these remote initiations were performed, or how the ritual of them differed from in-person or "live" ceremonies. For this reason, *shihan* are discouraged from attempting them. These remote initation practices are considered nonstandard at best, and downright preposterous by most. The *reiju* is a sacred

---

*Hawayo Takata is known to have occasionally initiated students who were not physically present. One such example is the American heiress Doris Duke. Takata trained her in the second degree via telephone and sent letters containing further notes and copies of the Reiki symbols. Although Takata-sensei was clearly capable of initiating students remotely, she only ever chose to do so "when the recipient was in the hospital or was far away and in obvious need. Clearly this way of teaching was the exception rather than the norm" (Fueston, *Reiki: Transmissions of Light,* 213).

ceremony, not one that should be taken lightly or entered into without adequate consideration and training.

The Inner Workings of Initiation

During an empowerment ceremony the *shihan* or instructor establishes a connection to the student and to Reiki itself. The teacher is nothing more than a conduit through which Reiki flows for the sake of bringing new practitioners into alignment with its source. Before this rite, the student is relatively unable to experience the inherent Reiki energy in his or her makeup; afterward he or she can sense and direct it instantaneously.

Mrs. Takata often made the analogy that the initiation process was much like fixing or upgrading a radio. She described herself as the master repairman, and the initiation itself as akin to fixing or changing the antenna in order to connect the student to the infinite wave of Reiki flowing through the entire universe.

Again, the initiation is sacred, so the details will not be provided here. Instead, know that the procedure itself enables the guiding consciousness of Reiki to adjust your energy field when you receive the *reiju.* It influences your aura, your meridians, and other aspects of your nonphysical being. Once the act is complete, Reiki will flow through your crown and down to the *hara* or lower *tanden,* an energy reservoir located just below your navel.

Whenever you practice Reiki, either for healing or in meditation, Reiki will initially fill this center. This is analogous to the charging of a battery. From there it flows upward toward the heart and out through the arms and hands. Reiki will also flow through the soles of the feet, out of the eyes, and with the breath. Because of this, during the initiation most traditions of Reiki will ask you to place your feet firmly against the floor, close your eyes, and hold your hands in *gasshō* (prayer position) to prevent any errant energy from leaking out.

With every additional attunement, the ability to transmit Reiki is refined. Takata described this as changing from 20 horsepower in the first degree to 100 horsepower in the second. Usui and Hayashi offered regular opportunities to refine practitioners' abilities through repeated *reiju,* a practice being reclaimed by some teachers today. Whether you are receiving your first or your tenth initiation, the essence of Reiki guides the process and assists you in recognizing your inherent wholeness.

Preparing for Your Initiation

There are many ways to prepare for your initiation prior to your Reiki class. If you approach the experience with reverence, you are likely to get more out of it. Since very few of us come from the same background as Usui-sensei, we cannot expect to have the spontaneous contact that led him to found the system of Usui Reiki Ryōhō. Evidence suggests that his earliest students probably underwent training in certain types of meditation or breathwork before they ever received their first *reiju.* Today this is seldom the case, given that Reiki students come from all walks of life and spiritual backgrounds.

Preparing yourself for your Reiki initiation can augment the energetic effects of the ceremony. Unlike Usui, we do not need to fast for three weeks straight, meditating day and night as we prepare to leave the earthly plane. Our founder created the *reiju* ceremony to empower students. Various branches of Reiki have altered or augmented the empowerment in order to enable students to receive a single transmission and still retain the ability to practice Reiki. Another way to enhance the efficacy of the initiation is to try out some of the following practices:

- Spend time in quiet reflection or contemplation.
- Consume as many fresh fruits and vegetables as possible.
- Increase your water intake.
- Eliminate or reduce stimulants, such as nicotine and caffeine.
- Reduce or eliminate consumption of alcohol.
- Spend less time watching TV, connecting to media (especially news programs), and on the computer or telephone.
- Invest time in healthy physical activity or in nature.
- Cultivate an attitude of gratitude, recite the Five Principles, meditate, or otherwise engage in a spiritual practice.[2]

This is by no means a comprehensive list of all the ways to prepare yourself to be a vessel for Reiki. It is also important to note that none of these steps is *required.* Engaging in healthy behaviors is an excellent practice, but making steps in the right direction can look different for each person. Remember that Reiki has no morality, and it offers no judgment for your actions. Only participate in the activities that are reasonable and attainable; if you've never fasted before, going on a juice cleanse won't make your Reiki class more enjoyable. In fact, it may do the opposite. Similarly, if you are a hard-core caffeine user, suffering from withdrawal isn't likely to help you stay focused during class.

Use your best judgment as to how you would like to prepare for your initiation. If nothing else, set aside time away from distractions in order to pray, meditate, or journal. Remember to reflect on the third Reiki principle: *kanshashite*—be grateful!

THE DEGREES OF REIKI

Reiki is taught in progressive degrees, which is one of the aspects common to all branches of it. The structure of Reiki teaching has evolved, even within the four years that Usui Mikao taught his healing art. Initially, Reiki Ryōhō lacked any formal structure. It was added in stages during and after Usui's years with the *gakkai.* In my own classes, I've chosen to use the most common Japanese titles for the three main levels of Reiki, for they convey a sense of what is learned in each seminar. Different branches of Reiki in Japan employ different names, with classes sometimes being offered in more than just three levels, much like Western Reiki.

Before beginning your Reiki training, it may help to familiarize yourself with what is offered at each level. This can help you decide how far you would like to take your training. Every level offers a unique set of tools; these tools empower you to heal on all levels of your being. Be sure to ask your teacher how many levels the three degrees are divided into in the branch of Reiki he or she is teaching. Three or four levels are the most common, but there are traditions offering seven or more.

Class format in each level is relatively similar for most branches of Reiki. Your teacher may prefer to maintain an oral tradition, or you may receive written and printed materials. Reiki history is conveyed, initiations are conferred, and hands-on practice is offered. Your teacher's style and personal connection to Reiki may also influence how the degrees are taught.

Historically, Reiki Ryōhō was offered in a slightly modified training format. Students were required to attend lectures prior to enrolling in the *shoden* course.[3] At one point, Usui numbered the levels of his system from six to one, in a manner consistent with degrees used in some Japanese martial arts: *roku-tō* (sixth level), *go-tō* (fifth level), *yon-tō* (fourth level), *san-tō* (third level), *ni-tō* (second level), and *ichi-tō* (first level). At a later stage he may have used a style similar to that of aikido.* Currently, the Usui Reiki Ryōhō Gakkai uses a means of dividing the degrees in a manner that is a compromise between them. The *shoden* degree consists of four parts (*roku-tō* through *san-tō*); *okuden* consists of two parts (*okuden zenki,* meaning "first part of *okuden,*" and *okuden kōki,* meaning "later part of *okuden*"), and finally there is *shinpiden,* the highest level taught.

Shoden (初傳)

The first degree is called *shoden* in Japanese. Its name means "first teachings" or even "entrance teachings." The first Reiki class for many people is an opportunity to open up and allow healing to enter their lives. Participants receive initiation, discuss the history of Reiki, learn the *gokai,* and practice the basics of treatment. *Shoden* places an emphasis on physical treatment and self-treatment, although first degree practitioners are certainly able to apply Reiki to a variety of circumstances and people.

In the level one class, different teachers will use different numbers of attunements or *reiju.* When Usui-sensei taught *shoden* it was broken down into four levels, which likely serves as the basis for Takata-sensei's

---

*This has not yet been verified, though more than one source has suggested it.

method of teaching the first degree class over four consecutive evenings.⁴ Students received an initiation with each progressive installment. Nowadays, other Japanese lineages, including Jikiden Reiki, still offer multiple *reiju* for the *shoden*-level students. Many other branches of Reiki have simplified their teaching style, and they provide one attunement for the first degree.

At the initial level of practice, new Reiki students are strongly encouraged to practice. The more you engage with your Reiki practice, the more sensitive you become to its use. Usui-sensei introduced the concept of *byōsen* (病腺) to his students at this level. *Byōsen* is spiritual blockage or disharmony, which produces sensations that practitioners experience when they give Reiki as a result of a state of energetic empathy. It is considered the cornerstone of level one practice, and Usui would not allow students to progress to *okuden* without having first learned to distinguish and treat the different levels of *byōsen.*

Since Usui Mikao initially adapted his journey toward *anshin ritsumei* as a spiritual practice, he incorporated the Five Principles into his teachings at level one. Rather than just being simple guidelines, they were meant to be tools for spiritual transformation. He encouraged his students to live by the *gokai,* and only those individuals who were committed to them were able to learn the higher degrees of Reiki.

Several additional techniques were included in the *shoden* classes. Usui provided simple measures to cleanse the practitioner's energy before and after treatment, as well as methods for connecting to Reiki and harnessing intuition for better and more accurate treatment. These methods have been recovered and reintegrated into many Takata-based lineages in the last couple of decades; collectively they are often referred to as the Japanese Reiki Techniques.

Naturally, practice makes perfect. To become a competent healer, Reiki practitioners have to practice. No amount of class time can take the place of personal practice. After the *shoden* class, Reiki is in your hands, literally. Take time each day to master the skills you've learned, and practice living by the Reiki Principles. As you focus on these aspects more and more, you will find that your ability to channel Reiki naturally increases.

Okuden (奥傳)

The second level of Reiki training means "inner teachings" in Japanese. *Okuden* was originally taught in two sections, with two *reiju* to accompany them. Mrs. Takata sometimes used only one initiation, and at other times two.[5] Second degree students are generally expected to have been diligent in their personal practice, thus mastering the foundation of Reiki treatments.

At the second level, Reiki practitioners are taught three symbols and their accompanying mantras/names. These symbols are regarded as sacred, and students are asked to show respect to the teachings by not openly displaying them or sharing them with individuals not initiated to the *okuden* level. The symbols are used to empower and specialize the flow of Reiki during a treatment; they will be discussed in brief below.

Level two classes are generally focused on the actual practice of Reiki. Class time should permit students to further their relationship with Reiki by exploring how to use the symbols in treatments and how to perform distance healing and psychological healing, as well as how to improve the strength and efficacy of treatments overall.

Usui-sensei also taught some additional techniques at the *okuden* level, many of which are meditative in nature. They help practitioners cultivate greater ki and strengthen their connection to Reiki itself. More Japanese Reiki Techniques are provided in the *okuden* class to ensure the personal and spiritual development of students.

Shinpiden (神秘傳)

Shinpiden means the "mystery teachings." This level is today known as the Master level or the Master/Teacher level. In lieu of a formal class structure, Usui's *shinpiden* students apprenticed beneath him until they mastered the ability to confer *reiju* and portrayed the spiritual qualities of the practice. Today, students are able to take a seminar over the course of a weekend in order to attain the degree of Reiki Master.

Shinpiden students were very rare in Usui Mikao's day; of the more than two thousand students he initiated into Usui Reiki Ryōhō, only approximately nineteen of them were teachers, accounting for less than

1 percent of his total students. He was clearly very selective with his future teachers, for they would be responsible for carrying the teachings into subsequent generations. Usui's intention was for Reiki to spread across the entire world. Thus he wanted to ensure that Reiki teachers would maintain the practice with integrity.

In modern branches of Reiki, the third degree is sometimes broken up into more than one class, enabling students to progress at a level they feel comfortable with as well as providing options for further training for those individuals who do not yet have the desire to teach. It is common for *shinpiden* to be divided into 3A and 3B (or sometimes 3 and 4), often called Advanced Reiki Training and Reiki Master/Teacher Training.

Even Japanese lineages have historically subdivided the teaching degree into several stages. Practitioners initiated into the mystery teachings would first become *shihan-kaku,* or assistant instructors/teachers, before graduating to the title of *shihan. Shihan-kaku* practitioners learn how to perform *reiju* and can teach only the first degree. *Shihan* are equivalent to Reiki Master/Teachers and permitted to teach the remaining levels. Some schools also delineate *dai shihan* ("senior instructor") as the only level capable of initiating other *shihan.*

At the Reiki Master level, students are expected to live by the Reiki Principles as best they are able, as well as to have committed themselves to regular practice on themselves and others. During training to become an instructor, students usually learn one more traditional Reiki symbol; some lineages have incorporated additional nonstandard symbols into this degree as well. The final symbol is used for initiations.

In addition to learning how to pass attunements, the practical matter of how to plan and deliver Reiki seminars is also a frequent component of *shinpiden* training. Many teachers prefer for students to co-teach or shadow several classes at the earlier degrees as part of their training. This apprenticeship method ensures consistent delivery and greater confidence during the new teachers' first classes.

Although the term *master* is frequently used in the West, it is entirely absent in traditional lineages in Japan. As Reiki instructors we do not master anything, except maybe our communication and teaching skills. It is an egoic mind that thinks it can master Reiki, for the spiritual truth is that sincere teachers allow Reiki to master them.

LINEAGE AND FORM OF PRACTICE

When you receive your first Reiki initiation, you aren't simply plugged into the spiritual, universal energy of Reiki; you also become a link in a chain that makes its way back through each generation of practitioners to the founder of Reiki Ryōhō, Usui Mikao. This succession of teacher to student is deemed to be one's "lineage." All authentic Reiki practices can trace their lineage back to Usui, although the length and complexity of lineage can sometimes be confusing.

No single lineage is considered more powerful or effective than any other. However, there are often significant distinctions between the styles and teachings of different lineages. Part of this is due to the nature of the oral tradition employed by seminal Reiki figure Takata-sensei, as well as her dynamic ability to present the material in such a way as to connect to the individuals in each class. After her passing in 1980, teachers eventually began to deviate from her teachings. Some added other spiritual topics and healing tools to their classes, whereas others radically changed the scope of the Reiki they taught.

Today we can celebrate the many ways that Reiki presents itself to the world and learn how to define our practice by better understanding the traditions and conventions of the Reiki system. Our lineage maps out where we are different, but it also invites us to recognize that each of us is descended from the spiritual awakening of Usui-sensei.

The Importance of Lineage

When selecting a teacher it's important to have access to his or her lineage to ensure that you are really learning an authentic branch of Reiki. And yet although lineage is important to the understanding of Reiki, it is nearly irrelevant to its application. In other words, the person you've learned Reiki from might shape your personal views of what Reiki is, but this has no bearing on your ability to practice healing or to grow through personal development.

Another layer of the significance of lineage can be better understood through the lens of a Japanese cultural worldview. The traditional arts in Japan such as flower arranging and the tea ceremony adhere to the teachings left by the great masters in their various lineages. These schools require developing students to closely follow the teachings of whoever established that lineage. The reason is not to create uniformity or suppress innovation. Paying homage to one's lineage provides a sense of continuity and adds context to one's practice, offering a stable platform for growth.

In the same fashion, learning about the teachers in one's lineage often plays a role in the *shoden* classes of most Reiki systems. We learn about the founder and his successors so that we can learn from their examples. Hawayo Takata, Yamaguchi Chiyoko, Hayashi Chūjirō, and Usui Mikao were all amazing teachers in their own right. By honoring our lineage we can preserve the contributions that each of them made to Reiki and to the Earth as a whole.

Duty and honor are important concepts in Japanese culture. When Takata-sensei taught the *gokai,* she often expanded them to include "honor your parents, teachers, and elders" because there is less emphasis placed on this in Western culture. (It is a given that you will respect your teachers and your elders in Japan.) In light of this, honoring your teacher means staying true to your lineage. When you create innovations in the Reiki system, do so in a way that respects the practice you've learned. Similarly, when you practice Reiki, remember to respect the way you have learned to do so. We all grow, and it is likely that we will leave some methods in the past, but that doesn't mean we throw them away once and for all; rather, we learn to honor how Reiki has helped us evolve so that we can strive for new things.

Common Styles of Reiki

There are dozens and dozens, perhaps even hundreds, of branches of Reiki practiced today. Some of these systems are clearly traceable to

Usui Mikao, while others seem a bit hazy in their lineages. To add to this confusion, instructors who study with more than one teacher may not disclose their entire lineage for the sake of simplicity. All of this leads to confusion about which elements are found in which branches of Reiki.

Usui called his practice Usui Reiki Ryōhō, or Shin Shin Kaizen Usui Reiki Ryōhō, and many teachers prefer to use this expression today. Takata referred to her practice as Usui Shiki Ryōhō, meaning "Usui-Style Healing Method." The *hanko* or seal she used on certificates actually names the system Usui Shiki Reiki Ryōhō, or Usui-Style Reiki Healing Method.[6] Many independent Reiki teachers use these names to describe what they teach also.

Reiki lineages may essentially be classified into four groups: traditional Japanese Reiki, traditional Western Reiki, hybrids of Japanese and Western Reiki, and nontraditional forms of Reiki.

The first group may be referred to as *dento Reiki* (傳統靈氣), meaning "traditional Reiki." Though this term is most commonly used to refer to the system of Reiki Ryōhō practiced by the Usui Reiki Ryōhō Gakkai in Japan, it can be extended to include other unaltered branches of Reiki that have evaded the process of Westernization. Other traditional styles of *dento Reiki* include Jikiden Reiki and the Reiki practiced as folk medicine throughout Japan. This latter style exists in several regions of the country, and it does not adhere to any standardized treatments nor belong to any organization. Several Reiki researchers, including Doi Hiroshi, Nishina Masaki, and Frank Arjava Petter, have documented examples of these practitioners, some of whom learned Reiki directly from Usui and his original *shihan*. All of the styles of traditional Reiki in Japan can trace their lineages through Usui and his group of nineteen *shihan*.

The second category of Reiki styles is that of traditional Western Reiki. Originally called Usui Shiki Reiki Ryōhō (later simply Usui Shiki Ryōhō or Usui-Style Healing Method), Western Reiki as it was taught by Hawayo Takata was adapted especially for Western audiences. Takata preserved many of the original concepts of *dento Reiki* while simplifying the overall structure of Reiki. Today, traditional Western Reiki lineages include those of the Reiki Alliance, early verisons of the Radiance Technique, and a number of independent teachers and practitioners who maintain practices nearly identical to those of Takata. All traditional forms of Western Reiki can trace their lineages through Hawayo Takata and her twenty-two *shihan.*

After Reiki was rediscovered in Japan in the 1990s, a number of teachers set out to bring together the best practices of both Eastern and Western lineages. (These have sometimes resulted in "reconstructionist" movements such as Usui Dō and Usui Teate, which aim to present themselves, rather misleadingly, as Usui's "original" teachings.) In any event, this third family of Reiki systems are those that combine the methodologies of both *dento* and Westernized Reiki practice. These are considered "hybrid" styles of Reiki in that they incorporate material from different lineages. They include:

- Gendai Reiki Hō
- Kōmyō Reiki Dō (formerly Kōmyō Reiki Kai)
- Vortex Reiki
- Reiki Jin Kei Dō
- Reido Reiki
- Seimei Reiki Ryōhō
- Usui Reiki Ryōhō, as taught by independent teachers and organizations such as International House of Reiki

There are also many Reiki systems that offer inaccurate or mythological lineages in an attempt to make their teachings seem more authentic, as with some of the reconstructionist movements mentioned above. These, too, can be considered hybrid forms of Reiki, for they offer information and practices from both Eastern and Western lineages.

Many other types of Reiki embraced innovation early on, adding on teachings such as information about chakras, the aura, meridians, crystals, color healing, and various other topics. These branches of Reiki often infuse the practice with a New Age flavor, and they may typically offer a single initiation per level. This fourth group is sometimes called nontraditional Reiki, though some practitioners prefer the term *evolved Reiki*. Such forms of Reiki sometimes have more complex lineages because they result from a combination of several lines into a single set of practices.

Some nontraditional branches commonly practiced are:

- Raku Kei Reiki
- Usui/Tibetan Reiki
- Radiance Technique (later versions)
- Rainbow Reiki
- Karuna Reiki
- Seichim, or Sekhem, Reiki
- Holy Fire Reiki
- Angelic Reiki
- Violet Flame Reiki
- Shamballa Reiki
- Kundalini Reiki
- Reiki Tummo
- Lightarian Reiki
- Ascension Reiki
- Blue Star Reiki

These systems of Reiki often make unverifiable or mystical claims about what sets their practices apart from other forms of Reiki Ryōhō, and they tend to misrepresent the history of Reiki (intentionally or not) to meet their own agendas. Many of the nontraditional forms of Reiki bear little resemblance to the other three categories of Reiki lineages.

It is important to recognize that a complete list of Reiki branches is virtually impossible to compile, for they continue to grow with each passing year, and an exhaustive list is outside the scope of this work. What matters is that the form of Reiki you learn and practice serves you and your healing journey. There are many teachers and practitioners who refer to their style as Usui Reiki, and many more independent teachers have *Usui Shiki Ryōhō* or *Usui Reiki Ryōhō* listed on their certificates. To better understand what form of Reiki your prospective teacher adheres to, ask him or her about lineage, how and when they learned it, and other pertinent details that would be helpful to know.

In a world where diversity is celebrated, we as Reiki practitioners need to find peace between our organizations and lineages. There is no need to feel that one type of Reiki is superior to any other, only that the form of practice it uses may be better suited to some individuals more than others. The many branches of Reiki Ryōhō are like the variety of ice cream flavors in the grocery store; not everyone will reach for the same one. As Reiki proliferated, it diversified in such a way that it is now able to reach more people, with each interested person being drawn to the practice that best meets the needs of their particular spiritual journey.

FINDING THE RIGHT TEACHER

Your choice of a Reiki teacher will impact your practice in numerous ways. For starters, the way he or she teaches will affect how you learn. If you are a hands-on learner, then you'll flourish with a teacher who emphasizes that aspect of the practice. Your lineage is also conferred through your teacher, so you will share a bond, just as you will with all Reiki practitioners—past, present, and future. Establishing a good relationship with the right teacher can help you take your practice to the next level, thereby enabling you to experience deeper healing with each part of your being.

Given that Reiki is learned in person, your teacher should be someone with whom you feel comfortable. He or she should be knowledgeable in the system and practice of Reiki. It is best to find someone with real-life experience with Reiki, not just someone who teaches without practicing outside the classroom. Ultimately, finding the right fit can make or break your Reiki practice. Below I provide some sample questions that you may ask your prospective *shihan* or Reiki Master in order to determine whether or not they are the perfect match for you.

How long have you practiced Reiki? How long have you taught?
What does Reiki mean to you?
What do you charge for classes? For treatments?
Can you give an example of how Reiki has helped you?
What led you to practice Reiki?
What system of Reiki do you teach?
Can you provide your lineage?
Do you engage in self-treatment?
Do you treat others?
Do you teach exactly what you learned, or have you made alterations/ changes?
Why do you teach Reiki?
What support do you offer to your students?
Do you use a manual in class? Which one?
How much practice time is offered in class?
What do the Five Principles/*gokai* mean to you?
What was your training like?

There is no definitively correct answer for each question, though some answers may raise red flags. For example, if someone cannot provide their lineage or doesn't remember the precepts, there's a good chance that their primary concern is not with the heart and soul of Reiki but just with its use in hands-on healing. If someone informs you that their own training was done online or through a DVD, you are unlikely to experience authentic Reiki no matter how sincere the practitioner may be.

Engage in an honest, transparent dialogue with your Reiki teacher-to-be. Perhaps you will find that you just don't click on a personal level, even though he or she may be a dynamic and effective teacher. Given that Reiki is such a profoundly personal, spiritual practice, you might opt for someone who better relates to you instead. Weigh each piece of information reasonably and do your research. You often get what you pay for, so find someone who offers excellent training for the right price.

Reiki Is the Real Teacher

At the end of the day, we all are connected to the same Reiki. The form of practice we use to tap into it may differ, but Reiki is our real teacher. Hawayo Takata was well known for her injunction, "Let Reiki teach you." Whoever goes through the physical ritual of initiation with you is just a facilitator; Reiki itself is the real source of the empowerment. Remember this when you are looking for the right teacher; Reiki will guide you.

You can't learn Reiki by reading about it, participating in academic seminars about it, or watching DVDs about it. That is part of what makes Usui Reiki Ryōhō so unique. The only genuine way to learn is through practice. Whatever method you are taught for harnessing Reiki in your life, there is no reward to be gained if you don't use it. Let your conscious mind and ego step away so that you can surrender to it. It will teach you through attunement and sensitivity; listen to your inner awareness as Reiki nudges you forward. As we learn to let go and listen to the same *dai Reiki* that awakened Usui Mikao on Mount Kurama, we will release our old hurts and gradually awaken to the truth of our inner divinity.

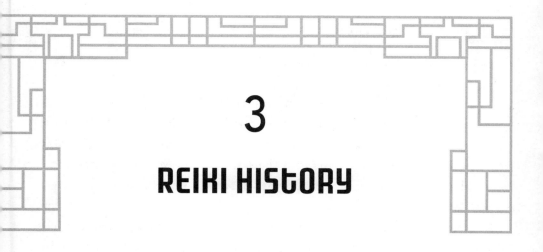

3

REIKI HISTORY

MANY CLAIMS ABOUT REIKI'S ORIGINS have been made in the last thirty years. If we were to believe them all, then Reiki would have originated in Tibet, Atlantis, Lemuria, or even another dimension altogether. There are researchers who asserted that Usui Mikao was a Buddhist of either the Tendai or Shingon schools, or even that he was Christian. Many other details about his life have been misrepresented, confused, and embellished, too. Some teachers have made culturally inaccurate assertions about the Reiki symbols and the methods of Reiki, and, as we have established, they have even added or deleted elements of traditional Reiki to support their cases. As more and more changes are made, the Usui System of Natural Healing has begun to lose a connection to its roots. An accurate depiction of Reiki history gives practitioners, teachers, and scholars a firm basis for understanding what Reiki really is.

WHY HISTORY MATTERS

Each year we piece together more about Reiki. And yet decoding the origins of Reiki and the life history of Usui Mikao has been slow going. Several factors, many of them relating to the passage of time, have inhibited the acquisition of a complete history of events. However, with growing participation among Reiki communities and laudable efforts by many valuable researchers and teachers, both

Eastern and Western, we are getting a clearer image of the genesis of Reiki as we know it.

For now I will attempt to summarize the main points in the history of Usui Reiki Ryōhō. It isn't entirely possible to include all of the research that's been conducted on Reiki, its founder, and the many teachers who have transmitted the system. However, as we learn more about Reiki's past, we can prepare ourselves for its future. Gaining a clear understanding of the origins of Reiki gives us context and understanding about what it is that we are practicing, as well as providing clear illustrations of what it does and does not offer. Furthermore, only by understanding the culture and practices of the origins of Reiki may we truly anticipate where Reiki will take us in the future.

There are three distinct periods in Reiki history: inception, transmigration, and globalization.[1] The phases are characterized in part by their geographical setting, and they overlap slightly. The period of inception takes place in Japan and begins in the 1800s prior to the formation of Usui Reiki Ryōhō; it includes the political and social reforms that gave rise to the new religious movements of the nineteenth and twentieth centuries. The second period is the North American era, which began when Hawayo Takata learned the system from Hayashi and started training others in Hawaii in the 1930s. Finally, the third period more or less began after the passing of Takata-sensei in 1980.

BUILDING A CONTEXT

As a whole, the earliest period in Reiki history reflects the original teachings of Usui Mikao with very few changes. This era emphasizes simplicity in its teachings, the importance of honoring lineage, and maintaining the integrity of the system. Although Usui Reiki Ryōhō didn't formally begin until after Usui's revelatory experience on Mount Kurama in March of 1922, the cultural climate of Japan in Usui's lifetime played a major part in the birth of Reiki.

Some background information on the history of Japan and its unique spiritual practices will be explored in brief below before diving into the life and merits of Usui. Although some of the events below may seem unrelated to Reiki, know that the unique society in which Usui lived is responsible for the way Reiki was created and shared, and it lives on in the forms of Reiki healing that are available today.

For Western audiences, a little background on Japan and its culture will broaden the appreciation and understanding of Reiki Ryōhō. Japan has historically been a place where the arts, philosophies, and influences of surrounding countries, such as China, Korea, and Russia, have transformed and syncretized with native ideologies. The end result is a way of life that is purely and uniquely Japanese. The cultural norms of Japan value tradition, simplicity, respect and honor, and a sense of belonging.

Japan is called *Nihon* or *Nippon* in Japanese, which is written as 日本 in kanji. This expression combines the words for "sun" and "origin" in a manner that more poetically translates as "Land of the Rising Sun." Apart from referring to Japan's geographic location in the Far East, it also illustrates the cosmology of Shinto, the native religion of Japan, which teaches that the act of Creation began with bringing the Japanese islands into existence.

Reiki is a Japanese art and it therefore embodies many of the traits of Japanese culture. Certain elements of Reiki, such as tracing one's lineage back to the founder and the practice of specific ideals (the *gokai*), emphasize its origins in the Land of the Rising Sun. Reiki Ryōhō stresses the importance of healing the *kokoro* both through the practice of the Five Principles and with hands-on healing. It also shares its roots with many other spiritual movements that emerged within the same time frame as Usui Reiki Ryōhō.

Belief Systems in Japan

Japanese worldviews provide a unique perspective largely as a result of the nation's long cultural history. Among these is an emphasis on refining the self through continual personal development, upholding the honor and duty owed to one's family and other close circles, and an innate sense of responsibility and respect for all life. Japanese religious practices typically seek harmony with nature, and they help humankind live in the flow of the universe.

The two major religious practices of Japan are Buddhism and Shinto. Prior to the arrival of Buddhism in the sixth century (C.E.), the native religion had no formal name. The native traditions of Japan have since been called *Shinto* or *kami no michi* (神道). *Shinto* means "way of the kami." The word *kami* (神) is usually rendered as *god* or *gods* in English, but *kami* can represent major deities with well-known names, histories, and personalities just as equally as it can refer to the local minor spirits or deified forces of nature. Shinto stresses the importance of the natural world and has its roots in the indigenous shamanic practices of early Japan.

Buddhism covers a wide range of traditions based upon the teachings or dharma of the historical Buddha, named Siddhartha Gautama. In the sixth century it arrived in Japan via Korea and has coexisted with Shinto since then. Buddhist practices teach the importance of the mind, promote the idea of reincarnation, and point us toward a state of enlightenment or salvation, which is attainable over many lifetimes. The major schools of Buddhism in Japan belong to Mahayana traditions, and they include Zen, Tendai, Shingon, Jōdo Shū, and Jōdo Shin Shū. Unlike many other branches of Buddhism, they stress the importance of the here and now, teaching adherents that enlightenment is attainable in this very lifetime.

In addition to the two major religious bodies of Buddhism and Shinto, there are modern religious and spiritual movements in Japan today, as well as foreign ones. Practices like *shugendō,* made up of a sect of ascetics practicing in sacred mountains, reach back into Japan's antiquity. Some of the other spiritual practices, however, emerged in the nineteenth and twentieth centuries, like Reiki, as original movements. Others were brought to Japan through renewed contact with the outside world after the Meiji Restoration.

The Meiji Restoration (1868–1912)

Prior to the reign of the Meiji emperor (明治天皇, Meiji Tennō), Japan existed as a feudal society essentially ruled by military leaders called shogun; they belonged to the Tokugawa clan. During this period of

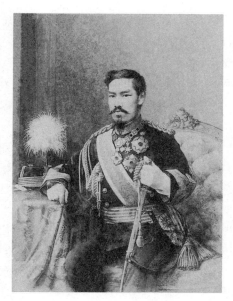

Emperor Meiji was a prominent nineteenth-century figure
whose leadership enhanced Japenese nationalism
and opened Japan to foreign trade and prosperity.
Portrait by Eduardo Chiossone, 1888

Japan's history, the country was closed off to foreign influences. When the Meiji emperor was installed as head of state in 1868, political power was consolidated under imperial rule. This had enormous impact on the social and political status of Japan.

The Meiji Restoration was responsible for rapid change and growth in all aspects of Japanese life. Reasserting the belief that the emperor was a direct descendant of the Shinto sun goddess Amaterasu Ōmikami resulted in a fierce rise in nationalism. This nationalism was now spiritual as well as social. The people were not merely believing in a political leader but in someone thought to literally be descended from the sun goddess. Emperor Meiji also reopened Japan's closed borders to promote foreign trade, which updated the beliefs and practices of its inhabitants. The heads of power during the restoration are responsible for having "stimulated [the] process of industrialization, modernization, the introduction of Western medicine and [the] Western school system."[2]

With a major shift in the cultural atmosphere of Japan, new spiritual movements blossomed rapidly. However, given the renewed integrity of imperial power and strict adherence to the national and spiritual imperatives to honor Shinto, many new traditions remained grounded in familiar practices, often by building ties to preexisting religions or honoring the emperor himself.

Emperor Meiji served as spiritual as well as political leader of Japan. He spearheaded the updating of a society that was far behind the rest of the world, and he did so without losing touch with his country's indigenous arts and traditions. Meiji Tennō is famed for having written upward of one hundred thousand traditional *waka* poems. *Waka* are characterized as having thirty-one syllables, and they often depict natural scenes and teach spiritual and moral lessons. The *waka* composed by the emperor are called *gyosei.* Usui Mikao admired Emperor Meiji greatly, and because of this he selected 125 of the emperor's poems as teaching tools in the *gakkai.*

New Religious Movements

The new religious movements began in 1814 with the founding of Kurozumi Kyō (a new religion largely derived from Shinto roots; founded in 1846), which would become a prototype of these kinds of movements. The majority of them were due to pervasive and increasing disillusionment with the Tokugawa shogunate (1600–1868), which was in its final years. Western spiritual thought was becoming more prevalent throughout the populace of Japan, with theosophy, New Thought, spiritualism, clairvoyance, mesmerism, and hypnotism representing some of the new spiritual practices available to Japanese people. Practices such as spiritualism "preserved or reanimated belief in the possibility of faith healing from modernization's rationalism."[3]

The new religious movements, called *shinshūkyō* (新宗教, or new sect teachings), were a reaction to the intellectual, rational, and "sanitized" mode of thinking that gave no room for the miraculous amidst everyday life. These new religious and spiritual groups were generally founded as offshoots of Shinto or Buddhism, making it possible for practitioners to follow the Japanese convention of upholding tradition. These movements typically exhibit very simple teachings and techniques, focus on benefits such as the possibility of salvation and healing, and introduce activities involving or benefitting others, such as healing or prayer.[4] Their expansion was closely monitored by the recently reformed Japanese government. Those systems that honored the emperor or developed out of State Shinto were often permitted to grow without concern. The *shinshūkyō* often maintained the belief in Japan as the origin of Creation, thus reasoning that the nation would be pivotal in the healing of the planet or the salvation of the human race.

Many of these organizations developed their own forms of healing, which harnessed a spiritually or divinely guided form of ki; examples of some of the terms coined for these styles of energy healing include:

- *seiki* (生氣)—vital energy, living energy
- *reishi* (靈子)—soul force, mysterious element
- *reiki* (靈氣)—soul energy, miraculous energy
- *jōrei* (浄靈)—purifying soul
- *yuki* (愉氣)—joyful energy, pleasant energy
- *kiai* (氣合)—uniting energy, usually featuring a short yell such as that released by martial artists

A small number of other schools practiced forms of healing with Reiki. Allegedly a twentieth-century Japanese therapist by the name of Kawakami Mataji created a form of practice that he called Reiki Ryōhō in 1914; however, this claim is disputed.* Several other spiritual schools taught forms of healing analogous to Reiki Ryōhō, such as Reikan Tōnetsu Ryōhō (靈感透熱療法), Senshinryū Reiki Ryōhō

---

*Founded in 1991, the International Center for Reiki Training, based in Southfield, Michigan, teaches several different styles of Reiki and offers certification programs in them. Although the center has, in the past, published information about Kawakami and a book he published on Reiki Ryōhō, no other researchers have been able to verify the claim that Kawakami Mataji created a form of Reiki Ryōhō. Indeed, in his book (*Reiki and Japan,* 32) Reiki *dai shihan* and researcher Nishina Masaki points out that no one else has yet been able to locate a copy of Kawakami's book.

(洗心流靈氣療法), and Seidō Reishōjutsu (生道靈掌術).[5] *Tenohira* or *teate* (healing by the laying on of hands) was a common element in these and other newly emerging healing modalities. In light of this, Usui named his system Shin Shin Kaizen Usui Reiki Ryōhō, or simply Usui Reiki Ryōhō, in order to differentiate from other varieties of Reiki therapy.*

By 1935 these new spiritual movements had reached their peak, having millions of adherents.[6] In a period marked by discontent, change, and uncertainty, individuals felt empowered by these emerging practices, and with them they learned how to heal and transform their lives. Although many of the smaller groups have disappeared, a handful spread as full-fledged religions, while others such as Reiki, Johrei, and Mahikari maintained their primary focus on healing and personal growth.

USUI MIKAO: FOUNDER OF REIKI

The founder of our system of Reiki Ryōhō is Usui Mikao. He was born in Taniai—a village in Gifu prefecture that lies west of the nation's current capital—on August 15, 1865.[†]

Usui-sensei was born into a family with ancient ties to the samurai; the Usui family has its origins in the Chiba prefecture to the north of Tokyo.[7] His father's name was Usui Uzaemon and his mother's was Kawai Sadako. Usui Mikao was the oldest of three brothers; the younger

---

*Bear in mind that Usui delineates that his system is entirely original. Although these other healing modalities included the expression *Reiki* in their names, they likely have no relationship with Usui's system of healing. There are some teachers and writers today who, in order to justify the significant changes they have made to their practice of Reiki, emphasize that Usui did not invent Reiki itself. Be mindful of this when seeking your own teachers; they should have an understanding of Reiki history and be able to present it without a bias that serves an egocentric agenda.

†Reiki researcher Justin Stein posits that Usui Mikao's actual date of birth was October 4, 1865, because the notation on his memorial stone (慶応元年8月15日, *keiō gan'nen 8-tsuki 15-nichi* [first year of Keiō period, eighth month, fifteenth day]) is representative of a non-Gregorian calendar common in Usui's day. Historians remain divided on both sides of this debate.

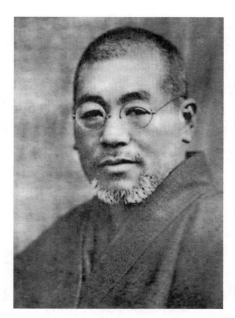

Usui Mikao,
the founder of Shin Shin Kaizen Usui Reiki Ryōhō

boys were named Sannya and Kuniji. He also had an older sister, Tsuru, but little is known of her.

In Usui Mikao's childhood, Taniai village had no school of its own so the local children received their education in the local temple, called Zendōji.[8] Zendōji is a Jōdo Shū (Pure Land) Buddhist temple, which confirms the sect that Usui belonged to, especially given that his remains are also interred in a Jōdo temple in Tokyo. Later in his youth, Usui Mikao would attend secondary school in a neighboring town.

Usui married and had two children. His wife's maiden name was Suzuki Sadako, and their children were a son, Fuji, and a daughter, Toshiko. Usui had a great number of professions, a detail hinted at on his memorial stone. Today we know through the dedicated work of Reiki researchers and teachers that Usui-sensei worked hard to achieve success and lasting happiness in several different fields, including work as a journalist, prison counselor, social worker, company employee, Shinto missionary, and public servant.[9]

Usui's professional life was quite abnormal among Japanese men, especially for the era in which he lived, given that the eldest son is expected to inherit the family business and care for his aging parents. Usui-sensei's decision to break free of these cultural expectations may have resulted in some family tension.* His middle brother, Sannya, became a doctor, and his youngest brother, Kuniji, took the reins of the Usui family business and cared for their parents.[10]

The founder of Reiki Ryōhō was the private secretary or *kaban mocha* (literally "briefcase carrier") to "one of the most outstanding politicians in modern Japan," a count named Gōto Shinpei.[11] Gōto had an illustrious and successful career, and during their time working together Usui built connections with officials in the government as well as in the army and navy. It is likely that Usui-sensei traveled to foreign countries as part of Gōto's retinue. After this period in his life, Usui branched out into business on his own, an endeavor that left him bankrupt at the age of fifty-five.

Usui-Sensei's Quest

This state of financial ruin led Usui to question his life's work and legacy. If each and every one of his forays into the professional world had failed, then he still had not achieved his life's purpose. Ultimately, this raised a fundamental question: What is the meaning of life? This contemplation compelled Usui toward achieving *anshin ritsumei* (安心立命), a state analogous to enlightenment, characterized by overflowing peace that enables attainment of one's destiny. Usui-sensei's memorial stone indicates that he studied many different spiritual practices, religions, and other esoteric tools along the way to uncovering Reiki Ryōhō.

The inscription on the Usui memorial describes the founder as being versatile, stating that he "loved to read books. He engaged himself in history books, medical books, Buddhist scriptures, Christian

---

*Usui's name is currently forbidden from being uttered aloud in the household of his descendants. The exact nature of the conflict is still unknown to researchers.

scriptures, and was well versed in psychology, Taoism, even in the art of divination, incantation, and physiognomy."[12] This great love of learning and his many areas of study paint Usui as a Renaissance man of his day, which breaks the convention of Japanese society. Most individuals of Usui's era apprenticed in a single school or art form and eventually became masters of their profession. The fact that Usui-sensei was atypical may have given him the unique perspective that led to the founding of his Reiki system of natural healing and spiritual growth.

Sometime around the year 1919, Usui began a three-year retreat at a Zen temple in Kyoto. Zen is one of the schools of Buddhism that focuses on the availability of enlightenment in the here and now. In his pursuit of *anshin ritsumei,* Usui most likely chose a Zen temple to experience a method of self-actualization that differed from the Buddhism of his family home. After three years, Usui still had not reached his awakening and asked the head of the temple for advice.

Having exhausted virtually every other means of awakening to *anshin ritsumei,* Usui was instructed by his teacher to try a more severe approach. In Japanese culture, certain ages are considered auspicious, while others are viewed as unlucky. In *mikkyō,* or esoteric Budhism, this translates to a belief that specific ages are windows for reaching enlightenment. Since Usui Mikao had passed the last of these windows, his Zen teacher suggested that he must prepare to die to attain enlightenment. Usui Mikao was told that sometimes when one is prepared to die, the flash of enlightenment becomes attainable. By approaching death by fasting and meditating, the soul may either prepare for one's next life to be one's final incarnation or less commonly the soul may be swept up by Amida Nyōrai and taken to the Pure Land, thus reaching enlightenment. Under this pretense, Usui-sensei made his way to a sacred mountain on the outskirts of Kyoto with the intention of fasting until he reached enlightenment—or perished trying.

Mount Kurama and the Birth of Reiki

In February of 1922 Usui Mikao climbed Mount Kurama in hopes of finding *anshin ritsumei.* In Takata's version of the Reiki origin story,

Usui meditated for twenty-one days, keeping track of time with a pile of small stones. The memorial stone inscription indicates that Usui spent approximately that length of time on the mountain, though it does not specify an exact number of days. And although we cannot determine with certainty the exact nature of his practice, Usui surely took advantage of the holy atmosphere pervading this mountaintop.

Kurama was home to a Tendai temple in Usui's time, although today a separate branch of Buddhism found only on this mountain, Kurama Kokyō, occupies this sacred land. Mount Kurama is also famed as the setting for a variety of Japanese myths and legends, many of which are fantastic in nature. It is a sacred space from top to bottom, with a unique mythology all its own. The mountain features waterfalls that are sometimes used in a purification ritual called *misogi* wherein the seeker stands beneath the falling stream of water in a meditative state to wash away sins and impure energies. Several authors have conjectured that this may have factored into Usui's practice on the mountain. More than likely, Usui Mikao simply meditated and fasted, preparing for the end of his life. It is unknown whether he performed any particular rituals, meditations, or mantra practices; whichever practices he pursued were likely only shared with his most advanced students and were probably never written down.

By the third week of fasting, Usui-sensei felt very weak and near death, and yet his ascetic practice paid off; he felt a *dai Reiki* (大靈氣), or great Reiki, over his head, which struck him like a great flash of light. Usui was rendered unconscious but the flash ushered him into a feeling of complete peace upon awakening, and he was refreshed and rejuvenated. The experience of receiving the flash of illumination, the great enlightenment, brought him back into a state of perfect health.

After this experience atop Mount Kurama, Usui summed up his experience of *anshin ritsumei* with the expression *uchū ware soku, ware soku uchū* (宇宙即我、即我宇宙). The kanji do not make for a good literal translation, but as we learned earlier in the book, this roughly means "you exist in the universe, and the universe exists in you."[13] In one sense this is a means of depicting the esoteric axiom "As above, so below," which implies that the macrocosm (the universe) and the microcosm (the self) are mirrors for one another. The *Reiki Ryōhō no Shiori,* a short booklet published in 1974 by the Usui Reiki Ryōhō Gakkai for its members, elaborates by stating that the small universe (the self) must become totally aligned with the spiritual power of the entire universe.[14] Doing so will confer a certain power to influence nature, such as through the healing gifts of Reiki Ryōhō.

Usui is said to have experienced several miracles upon leaving his retreat atop the mountain. The first occurred on his descent. Usui stubbed his toe, perhaps on one of the many cypress roots, and tore back his toenail. His natural instinct, which he followed, was to grasp the injury in order to staunch the bleeding; within moments he noticed that the pain had receded. When he inspected his toe, the nail had repaired itself and the blood had stopped flowing. This was his first experience with the miraculous power of Reiki. Although he had set out to attain *anshin ritsumei,* our founder had also received the ability to heal.

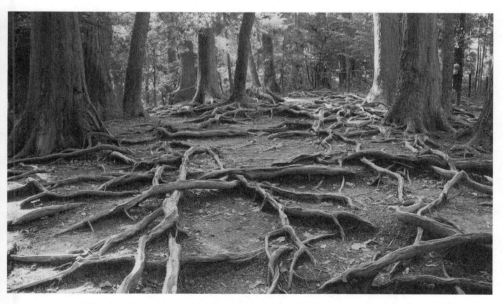

The landscape atop Mount Kurama in Japan, featuring what may be the very same roots that Usui tripped over when he first experienced the healing power of Reiki.

In the popular versions of Reiki history propagated by Western-derived lineages of Reiki, Usui is thought to have stopped at a local eatery or inn to break his fast. The owner of the facility could tell by Usui's haggard appearance that he had been in seclusion on the mountaintop for weeks, and he offered him a gentle meal preferred by most people returning from such ascetic practice. Usui-sensei, however, insisted on a hearty meal instead, and the innkeeper was amazed that Usui's stomach, thanks to Reiki, could tolerate it.

The kindly man who prepared Usui's food sent his granddaughter to deliver it to Usui. He noticed that she was in great pain, with tears streaming down her face. Upon inquiring why she cried, Usui learned that she had been suffering from toothache; the young girl was unable to visit the dentist for he was too far away. Usui compassionately offered to try his newfound Reiki gift on her, and the girl's pain dissipated altogether.

Thereafter, Usui returned to Kyoto to meet his teacher at the Zen temple. The teacher confirmed that the experience on Mount Kurama had indeed inaugurated *anshin ritsumei* and brought Usui the state of enlightened peace he had sought. Usui's teacher was also the first person to plant the seed for pursuing the healing arts, as he encouraged Usui-sensei to share this new gift with the world. Because *anshin ritsumei* is a deeply rooted peace that enables one to live out one's life purpose, upon his awakening to enlightenment, the gift of healing revealed itself to be Usui's particular purpose. He returned home to Tokyo and shared his newfound healing abilities with his friends and family. At this point, Usui formally incorporated his teachings into the practice named Shin Shin Kaizen Usui Reiki Ryōhō.

Usui Shares Reiki with Others

Usui is said to have had over two thousand students in the years between his awakening on Kurama and his death in 1926. In April of 1922, just one month after his experience on Kurama Yama, Usui Mikao founded the Usui Reiki Ryōhō Gakkai, or 臼井靈氣療法学会, in Japanese. This organization was based in Aoyama, Harajuku, in central Tokyo, not far from Meiji Jingu, the shrine commemorating Emperor Meiji. The *gakkai* served as his dojo, or training facility. As he shared his spiritual teachings, they became more codified and standardized in order to facilitate the learning process. Initially, Usui's method of healing and personal development had no normal name, no organized syllabus, and no ritual of initiation. New practitioners received *reiju* by merely spending time in Usui's presence or by listening to him recite the Meiji emperor's poetry.

In time, news of Usui's spiritual gifts and healing abilities spread far and wide. He endlessly gave Reiki treatments and eventually added the familiar concepts of the *gokai,* initiation ritual (*reiju* or attunement), and even the symbols and mantras taught in higher degrees of Reiki. In 1923, Tokyo was devastated by the Great Kanto Earthquake; Usui responded by serving those impacted by its destructive influence. Over one hundred thousand individuals died or went missing; even more were left injured or homeless.

At the time of the earthquake, Usui's previous employer Gōto Shinpei was mayor of Tokyo. Gōto organized aid for his citizens, and it is possible that he invited Usui to offer Reiki to survivors. Given that hospitals were also destroyed in the wake of the earthquake, officials relaxed the regulations around spiritual healers and encouraged them to help. According to one Japanese writer and researcher, Usui initiated several others as teachers of Usui Reiki Ryōhō in order to meet the great need for healing at that time.[15] This event sparked the spread of his Reiki system.

Practitioners in Japan claim that he would treat up to five people at once: one with each hand, one with each foot, and another still with his eyes and breath. It is estimated that thousands of individuals received healing from Usui and practitioners of his Reiki Ryōhō. This selfless act may have ignited the desire of many others to learn the system.

In the next few years Usui-sensei would move his teaching headquarters to a larger facility and begin to travel more frequently in order to teach Reiki across Japan. The *gakkai* grew very rapidly, in part due to his political connections. The Japanese Navy became familiar with Reiki, and several high-ranking officers brought it on board naval ships as a first aid measure and to reduce the amount of medical equipment necessary.

Usui's training center finally came to be located in Nakano, which was on the outskirts of Tokyo at the time. His travels continued, and on one of these teaching trips Usui-sensei experienced a stroke and ensuing cerebral hemorrhage. He passed away on March 9, 1926, in Fukuyama. Usui's ashes are interred at Saihōji in Tokyo, a Jōdo temple. At the time of his passing, there were over forty branches of the *gakkai* in Japan.[16] He was succeeded as president of the Usui Reiki Ryōhō Gakkai by Ushida Juzaburō. Subsequent heads of the society were Taketomi Kan'ichi, Watanabe Yoshiharu, Wanami Hōichi, Koyama Kimiko, Kondō Masaki, and Takahashi Ichita, who is still currently president.

PRESIDENTS OF THE USUI REIKI RYŌHŌ GAKKAI

NAME	TERM	LIVED
Usui Mikao (臼井甕男)	1922–1926	1865–1926
Ushida Juzaburō (牛田 従三郎)	1926–1935	1865–1935
Taketomi Kan'ichi (武富 咸一)	1935–?*	1878–1960
Watanabe Yoshiharu (渡辺 義治)	?–?	?–1960
Wanami Hōichi (和波 豊一)	?–1975	1883–1975
Koyama Kimiko (小山 君子)	1975–1998	1906–1999
Kondō Masaki (近藤 正毅)	1998–2010	1933–2010
Takahashi Ichita (高橋 一太)	2010–present	?–present

*As indicated by the question marks, some details about the dates of the lives and terms of the individuals listed above remain to be verified. For detailed biographical information, please see *This Is Reiki* by renowned Reiki author Frank Arjava Petter. For more on the information contained in this table, please see Mochizuki and Kaneko, *Chō Kantan Iyashi no Te*; Petter, *This Is Reiki*; and Doi, *A Modern Reiki Method for Healing*.

REIKI AFTER USUI

Usui trained other *shihan* who continued to propagate Reiki in Japan. In the four years between attaining *anshin ritsumei* and his death, Usui Mikao initiated over two thousand students. Less than 1 percent of them achieved the level of *shinpiden* and were able to spread Reiki Ryōhō after Usui's death. When Ushida-sensei, the second president of the *gakkai,* took his turn in leading practitioners of Usui Reiki Ryōhō, he made several reforms in an attempt to instill more structure into the practice.

Typically when a spiritual movement is in its inception phase, the structure and organization of the system tend to be fairly loose. The central figure in a movement, such as the founder or key teacher, is a living embodiment of the teachings; he or she *is* the structure. The same idea held true for Reiki. When Usui Mikao lived and taught, the organizational structure was fairly relaxed. He evaluated the skills of his students himself and permitted individuals to advance as their practice improved. There was no set curriculum for the third degree, or *shinpiden* teachings; instead, students would sit in on lectures with Usui until he deemed that they were ready to begin passing *reiju* to new members.

Considering this, Ushida Juzaburō chose to codify the teachings and techniques in the *gakkai*. Some researchers have speculated that his military background was a strong influence on his desire to delineate and control the structure of the *gakkai*. He helped develop a specific curriculum for each level of Reiki. This curriculum consisted of specific techniques (such as the Japanese Reiki Techniques introduced in later chapters) and ample practice.

Among the *shihan* were a number of other Japanese naval officers. Prior to Usui's death, his reverence and respect for the imperial system of Japan most likely prevented Reiki from being targeted by the strict legislation that arose to govern the new religious movements and alternative methods of healing.

Although the political ties that Usui had made working for Gōto

Shinpei continued to benefit the system of Reiki throughout his life, with the Meiji Restoration in 1868 came Western medicine and Usui Reiki Ryōhō was not among the practices legally permitted under the reformed government. The only traditional forms of medicine sanctioned under the reformed Japanese government were acupuncture and shiatsu, and practitioners of these modalities underwent strict certification. The members of the Usui Reiki Ryōhō Gakkai chose to close themselves to the public and reserve their practice for themselves and their families rather than contend with attempting to find a means to practice openly. After World War II, this became increasingly more difficult; many branches, including that of Usui's youngest brother Kuniji, closed.

Furthermore, after the end of World War II a regular meeting of former navy officials in Usui's organization would have been suspicious. Several of the presidents of the *gakkai* after Usui had been part of the navy, including Ushida Juzaburō. He is responsible for Usui's memorial stone and is the calligrapher behind the well-known version of the *gokai* that is available to us today.

There were nineteen *shinpiden*-level students who were given Usui's blessing to instruct others as *shihan* in the *gakkai*. Seasoned *okuden* practitioners led meetings and performed the monthly *reiju* at the branches' gatherings when there was no *shihan* available.[17] Although many members continued to practice in secret, some individuals chose to leave the *gakkai* for mostly unknown reasons. Among these were famed Japanese healer Eguchi Toshihiro and Tomita Kaiji, Reiki student and author of the book *Reiki To Jinjutsu—Tomita-ryu Teate Ryōhō.**

Eguchi disagreed with the high fees required for Reiki training with the Usui Reiki Ryōhō Gakkai, so he began to propagate his own

---

*Neither Eguchi nor Tomita were *shihan* in the Usui Reiki Ryōhō; it is believed that they were *okuden,* or second degree, practitioners. There is evidence that some *okuden* practitioners were shown how to perform *reiju,* especially in remote branches of the *gakkai* that may have lacked a *shihan.* It is possible that Eguchi and Tomita may have been familiar enough with performing *reiju* to develop their own forms of it.

system of healing, called Tenohira Ryōji (掌療治, or palm healing). Eguchi's organization is believed to have taught approximately five hundred thousand students.[18] Tomita called his modality Teate Ryōhō (手当療法, or laying-on-of-hands healing method), and his institute had over two hundred thousand students.[19] Both men made significant changes to Usui's system of Reiki Ryōhō, and they offered their teachings under new names accordingly.

Most practitioners of Reiki from Western lineages initially believed that *dento Reiki* had died out in Japan altogether. Likely due in part to the *gakkai's* exclusivity and secrecy, Reiki remained relatively unknown outside of small circles until it was rediscovered in Japan in the 1990s. In addition to the Usui Reiki Ryōhō Gakkai, some families preserved the Reiki teachings that they had learned from Usui's *shinpiden*-level teachers.

Hayashi Chūjirō

Arguably the most influential of Usui Mikao's Reiki *shihan* was a former navy captain named Hayashi Chūjirō. Hayashi was born on September 15, 1880. He enrolled in the Japan Naval Academy in 1899 and graduated three years later at the age of twenty-two.[20] He attained the rank of captain and worked in logistical positions at harbors, rather than on battleships on the front line. Hayashi and his wife had two children: a son, Tadayoshi, born in 1903, and a daughter, Kiyoe, born in 1910. Beginning in 1902, Hayashi-sensei spent four years serving in the Russo-Japanese War. In 1918, Hayashi Chūjirō was appointed director of Ominato Port Defense Station, at the foot of Mount Osore on the Shimokita Peninsula of northern Japan.[21] It was here that he would work with rear admiral Taketomi Kan'ichi; Taketomi may have introduced Hayashi to the system of Reiki, as he would become one of Usui's successors and the third president of the Usui Reiki Ryōhō Gakkai.

Most branches of Reiki, both Eastern and Western, claim that Hayashi was a medical doctor or a surgeon. Although definitive proof remains to be published, the Jikiden Reiki Kenkyukai asserts that they

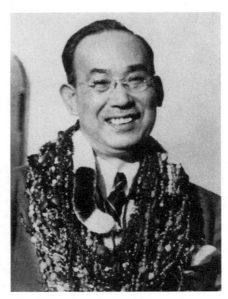

Hayashi Chūjirō was an important figure
in the history and growth of Reiki.

have found tax records indicating that Hayashi was indeed a medical
doctor, with a medical practice, at one stage in his life.*

Hayashi met Usui Mikao at a lecture on Reiki Ryōhō sometime
around 1924.[22] Hayashi, like several other officers of the navy, would
go on to study with Usui; he became a *shihan* in 1925. As one of the
last *shinpiden* students of Usui, a number of researchers have speculated, Hayashi may have received updated or modified teachings. It is
also true that Usui may not have completed his apprenticeship with
Hayashi. Since *shinpiden* means "mystery teachings," an incomplete

---

*Researchers Robert Fueston and Jojan Jonker both indicate that the title of *doctor* may
refer to an achievement other than medical doctor when applied to Hayashi. He was not
trained in medical sciences during his time at the naval academy but may have had extensive
training in hygiene and first aid. It is possible that Takata called him Dr. Hayashi because
of his extensive experience treating clients at his clinic. The Jikiden Reiki Kenkyukai claims
that Hayashi was a doctor, but no documents have been found to prove this definitively
just yet. Perhaps he received training in complementary or traditional medical practices,
such as traditional Chinese medicine, in addition to his Reiki training, later in life.

study may account for the less overtly spiritual and more clinical focus of Hayashi's teachings.

Due to Hayashi's purported medical background, Usui urged Hayashi to open his own dojo and teach Reiki through his more clinically minded perspective. Hayashi Chūjirō continued to practice and teach through the *gakkai* until he founded the Hayashi Reiki Kenkyukai in 1930, the same year that he retired as a naval captain and became a reservist.[23] He finally left the *gakkai* amicably in 1931, choosing to focus on his own school instead.

Dr. Hayashi updated the system of Reiki in several ways. First, his focus was predominantly on physical healing, or at the very least on the physical effects of healing through the spiritual gifts of Reiki. This may have been due to the navy's involvement in the early days of Reiki, given that they would have been less interested in the spiritual aspect of attaining *anshin ritsumei*. Hayashi also adopted the practice of using tables on which to give Reiki, much as we practice Reiki on massage tables today. He preferred for clients to be treated by two practitioners simultaneously, thus improving the efficacy of treatments at his clinic.

The cost of training was high in Hayashi's time; he often taught *shoden* and *okuden* together for the equivalent of approximately two months' salary. This enabled new students to hasten their study, obviating years of practice for the student before he or she could advance to the *okuden* class.

Reiki was regarded as a desirable trait for women seeking to start families, and in part for this reason Hayashi's classes were always full. Today, authentic Hayashi-style Reiki is still taught by the Jikiden Reiki Kenkyukai and is extant in some aspects of Usui Shiki Ryōhō as originally taught by Hawayo Takata.

Hayashi died in 1940, on May 11. He chose an honorable method of death by suicide as a means of avoiding conflict in the upcoming war. It is likely that Hayashi, having just returned from training practitioners in Hawaii, was pressured into revealing intelligence to the Japanese Navy, and this conflicted with Hayashi's otherwise peaceful way of life. In lieu of disappointing his country or causing harm to his students, Hayashi made his choice of death by suicide in accordance with Japanese culture and tradition, as a means of dying with honor. His wife, Chie, maintained the Hayashi Reiki Kenkyukai and served as president for the remaining years that it operated.

EAST MEETS WEST: TAKATA'S INFLUENCE ON REIKI

In the year 1935 the course of Reiki's history would be forever altered when Hawayo Takata, an American-born woman and the daughter of Japanese parents, traveled to Tokyo. She made her journey to tell her parents of her sister's recent passing and to seek medical treatment for a variety of conditions. According to the popular story she told, just as Takata was about to undergo anesthesia for surgery, her intuition guided her to seek an alternative treatment. This is how she was pointed in the direction of Hayashi's clinic.

Takata was born on the island of Kauai, in Hawaii, on December 24, 1900; she was considered to be nisei, or second-generation Japanese. Born as Hawayo Hiromi Kawamura, she was the daughter of Japanese immigrants who had moved to Hawaii to start their family. Hawayo worked hard, even early in life, and eventually began a family of her own after marrying Saichi Takata in 1917. Saichi died of lung cancer in 1930, leaving Takata to care for their two daughters, Julia and Alice.[24] Within five years, she developed gallstones, asthma, appendicitis, and at least one tumor as a result of her exhaustion.[25]

In 1935 Takata's sister died of influenza while her parents were visiting family in Japan. This was when Hawayo Takata seized the opportunity to travel to Japan to both inform her parents of her sister's untimely death and to take care of her medical concerns. She often recounted that while lying on the operating table, "[she] heard a voice inside her saying, 'This operation is not necessary.'"[26] When she asked her doctor for an alternative route of treatment, he asked his sister to take Takata to Hayashi-sensei's clinic.

Although this is the commonly accepted story, recent evidence

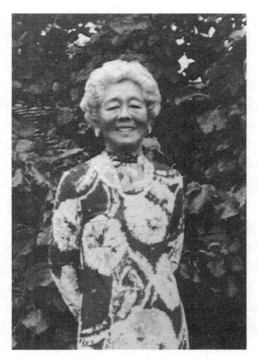

Hawayo Takata, whose encounter with Reiki would change
the course of Reiki history

may point to an alternative path by which Takata discovered Reiki. An
article published in the *Hawaii Hochi,* a Japanese-language newspaper
in Hawaii, indicates that prior to Takata, several other individuals in
Hawaii had learned Reiki from Hayashi-sensei. An article in that peri-
odical, dated September 30, 1937, states that Mr. and Mrs. Higuchi
from Hilo and a Mr. Tahara received instruction from Hayashi in
1933, two years before Hawayo Takata would visit Hayashi's clinic in
Tokyo.*[27] This article also reports that Takata studied with the Hayashi
Reiki Kenkyukai, stating, "Long ago, Mrs. Takata received a correspondence course [通信講習, *tsūshin kōshū*] from the Kenkyukai in Tokyo"

---

*Interestingly, Mr. Higuchi Kan was a pastor in Hilo, and Mr. Tahara Hiroshi was the
head of a Japanese school five miles outside of Hilo. Together, their occupations resemble
Takata's embellished depiction of Usui Mikao as a minister and head of a boys' school in
Kyoto in the version of Reiki pseudo-history that she told in her classes.

and that she visited Japan to further her training.[28] It is of special interest that the term *tsūshin kōshū** (通信講習) was used to describe her initial instruction; it may tell us that Takata fulfilled a prerequisite course before enrolling in *shoden* and *okuden* in Japan. This may have been analogous to the *roku-to* and *go-to* lectures that Usui required his prospective students to attend before entering the *shoden* seminar. I suspect that if Takata did indeed take a correspondence course in any form, it may have been intended to confirm her level of interest and commitment to Reiki.

However it was that Takata was introduced to Reiki, she was treated daily at Hayashi-sensei's clinic in Shinanomachi and within four days experienced a healing breakthrough. At that point, her gallstones were flushed from her system. Treatment nonetheless continued for weeks, after which time the popular version of Reiki history tells us that she plotted a way to learn Reiki. Initially her request had been refused by Hayashi because she would be returning to Hawaii, and although she was of Japanese descent, she was not a native-born citizen. (Reiki was esteemed and preserved as a uniquely Japanese art form.[†])

Takata as Apprentice

With the help of her friend and physician Dr. Maeda, Hawayo Takata eventually persuaded Dr. Hayashi to teach her Reiki.[29] After receiving approval from other *shinpiden* practitioners, Takata was offered training in *shoden* and *okuden*. Following months of treatment, Takata left Tokyo to attend to some family business. Upon returning, the Hayashi family invited Takata to live with them and continue her education.[30]

---

*Reiki teacher and researcher Nishina Masaki ("Hayashi's Activities in Hawaii," http:// jikiden-reiki-nishina.com/hawaii/) notes that the term *tsūshin kōshū* may in fact be used in error in the *Hawaii Hochi* newspaper. He reasons that there are numerous errors and typos throughout many of the articles and advertisements regarding Reiki and he posits that the journalist may also have recorded Takata's story incorrectly.

†Recent research has proved, however, that Hayashi apparently had no qualms about offering training in Reiki Ryōhō to outsiders, as there were already Reiki practitioners in Hawaii by 1933, when Takata visited his clinic.

She spent the next six months as Hayashi's prime pupil, studying Reiki with great enthusiasm.

Although to most Westerners this appears to be of little importance, Takata's invitation to live with her teacher granted her special status and enhanced access to the valuable training offered by Hayashi-sensei. In Japan a student who lives with his or her teacher for the express purpose of special training is called *uchideshi* (内弟子, or inside student).[31] This is considered to be a tremendous honor, one reserved for a select number of pupils. Becoming Hayashi's *uchideshi* afforded Takata the opportunity to learn at an accelerated rate, and she continued to work in his clinic and make house calls for patients unable to travel.

By May of 1936, Takata was studying *shinpiden,* or the third degree.[32] This enabled her to teach *shoden,* which she began to do upon her return to Hawaii later that year. She opened a clinic as a means of treating others with Reiki thereafter as well. Takata returned to Japan in 1937 for additional training and appears to have been granted permission to teach the beginning levels of Reiki Ryōhō. After returning to her home in Hawaii, Takata-sensei initiated approximately fifty new practitioners in her classes, and these students officially joined the Hayashi Reiki Kenkyukai.[33]

In October of 1937, Hayashi and his daughter Kiyoe arrived in Hawaii. Hayashi-sensei taught fourteen Reiki seminars, attended by approximately three hundred students; his daughter offered lessons in flower arranging and the tea ceremony. More than seventy articles, advertisements, and announcements were published in the *Hawaii Hochi* during the time that Hayashi visited and shortly thereafter. A certificate was issued in English for Takata on February 21, 1938, naming her "one of the thirteen fully qualified as a Master" in the art of teaching and transmitting Usui Reiki Ryōhō to others.[34]

The exact degree and title conferred to Takata during her time with Hayashi-sensei in Japan is currently contested, however. Robert Fueston, Reiki teacher and founder of the Reiki Preservation Society, believes that Takata was a fully fledged *shihan* by the time she left Hawaii, and that her English-language certificate confers the status of *dai shihan* (senior instructor) to her. He articulates this in his book *Reiki: Transmissions of Light.* Nishina Masaki, on the other hand, supposes that Takata was in fact only *shihan-kaku* (assistant instructor) upon her return to Hawaii, thus making her English-language certificate the equivalent of *shihan.*

Although copies of Takata-sensei's Master certificate are widely available, the Japanese-language certificates have not been made public. They are currently in the Takata archives, maintained by the Reiki Alliance and Takata's family. The exact reason that they have been withheld is not known, though personal reasons have been cited. In today's world these certificates, like any other historial document, can easily be amended or forged. Indeed, this has happened in the past in the case of other claims pertaining to the history of Reiki. Another possible explanation for their being withheld is that if Nishina's theory that Takata never received the title of *dai shihan* is correct, the certificates would provide evidence contrary to Takata's narrative.

Prior to Hayashi's arrival in Hawaii the term *Master* had never been used in relationship to Reiki. It appears that it was only adopted in English as indicated on Takata's certificate. I suspect that the wording on her Master certificate was chosen, or at least translated, by Takata herself. The earliest use of the term *Master* occurs only once prior to the issuing of Takata's certificate. The passenger manifest of the ship that Hayashi-sensei and his daughter Kiyoe boarded, the *M. S. Chichibu Maru,* lists Hayashi Chūjirō's occupation as Master of Hayashi Reiki Kenkyu.*[35] In this instance, I believe that *Master* may mean something more like *Headmaster,* as Hayashi was the leader and head teacher of the institute. It is possible that this official document may represent the beginnings of the term *Reiki Master.*

Hayashi Reiki Kenkyukai in Hawaii

After spending nearly five months in Hawaii, Hayashi Chūjirō had taught *shoden* and *okuden* fourteen times. He used the same five-

---

Kenkyu is used in lieu of *Kenkyukai* on the manifest because of limited space in which to write (on the manifest). It's interesting to note that on the original document, the handwritten words *spiritual healer* were added to this space, probably for clarification.

day format that Reiki teacher Yamaguchi Chiyoko would participate in soon after Hayashi's return to Japan (see page 80). Articles in the *Hawaii Hochi* indicate that during these classes, Hayashi welcomed approximately 350 new members to the Hayashi Reiki Kenkyukai.[36] On January 10, 1938, a formal branch of the Hayashi Reiki Kenkyukai opened in Hawaii. Hawayo Takata is listed as the sole *shihan* of the branch, and several other key roles have also been identified by Nishina Masaki, including treatment manager Aoyama Bunki, secretary Tamayose Hōun, and treasurer Ueda Masaichi. The head office of the Hawaii branch was located in the Globe Hotel.

Takata-sensei continued to deliver the *shoden* and *okuden* training on an almost weekly basis for some time after Hayashi's departure. Advertisements for these classes in the *Hawaii Hochi* name the system Usui Reiki Ryōhō, thereby indicating that no significant changes had yet been made in the process of transmigration. It is not presently known how many classes Takata gave before adapating Reiki Ryōhō. Initially, the majority of Takata's students belonged to the Japanese community in Hawaii, though there is some anecdotal evidence to suggest that she may also have taught on the West Coast of the United States. No evidence of her activities during World War II remains, which probably indicates that she suspended her classes to avoid unwanted attention from American authorities.

Reiki researchers Justin Stein and Hirano Naoko interviewed a few of Takata's earliest students. These were Reiki practitioners who belonged to the Japanese community of Hawaii. They are quite elderly now, given that they were Takata's pupils in the 1940s and 1950s. Stein and Hirano record that Takata

> never spoke of "universal energy," but rather of *reiki, meinai chikara* [見えない力] ("invisible power"), or *seishin no chikara* [精神の力] ("spiritual power"). One woman we spoke with, Yoshie Kimura, was initiated along with her parents during Takata's first class in Hiloin 1938. Regarding *uchū*, she said that Reiki taught that "the universe is as I am; I am as the universe is" (*uchū ware soku, ware soku uchū*

(宇宙即我、即我宇宙]), which she related to the expression "direct spirit" (*choku rei* 直靈), associated with one of the symbols taught to advanced practitioners.[37]

In this passage, the expression *uchū ware soku, ware soku uchū* echoes Usui-sensei's revelation upon attaining *anshin ritsumei*. Takata-sensei clearly learned this maxim from Hayashi himself, and she chose to impart it to her Japanese-speaking students during her first phase of teaching Reiki. All the evidence about Takata's classes in those days indicates that she delivered the same training that Hayashi did.

It is worth noting that contrary to popular belief, Hawayo Takata was not the only Reiki teacher in the West prior to 1976. Reiki researcher Justin Stein discovered that a Mr. Nagao Tsukuji and his daughter, having first studied Reiki with Takata in Hawaii, traveled to Japan to study *shinpiden* with Hayashi Chie, Hayashi-sensei's wife.[38] When the Nagao family was interviewed about Reiki, the descriptions of their treatments exactly matched the style taught by Hayashi (and therefore are also identical to those of the Jikiden Reiki Kenkyukai today). Although Mr. Nagao became *shihan* (or possibly *shihan-kaku*) in the 1940s, there doesn't seem to be much evidence that he contributed to the spread of Reiki in Hawaii.

Usui Shiki Ryōhō

Over time, the system of Reiki began to adapt to Western culture. When Hawayo Takata began teaching English-speaking audiences, the certificates she issued bore the name Usui Shiki Ryōhō (臼井式療法), or Usui-Style Healing Method.* The exact reason for the change is not

---

*A growing group of practitioners prefer the title Usui Shiki Reiki Ryōhō (臼井式靈氣療法), or Usui-Style Reiki Healing Method, for Takata's system of Reiki Ryōhō as it explicitly indicates that it is a healing method using Reiki. Usui Shiki Reiki Ryōhō also appears in an advertisement for Hayashi-sensei's seminars in Hawaii in the *Hawaii Hochi* in October 1937, perhaps to distinguish Hayashi's teachings from those of the Usui Reiki Ryōhō Gakkai (Nishina, "Hayashi's Activities in Hawaii," http://jikiden-reiki-nishina.com/hawaii).

known, although it reflects that several minor changes were made to Reiki as Takata taught it. The differences are mostly stylistic, and they enabled Reiki to flourish in the American culture.

The primary changes made to Reiki included the removal of Japanese terms. Many of the Japanese Reiki Techniques were still taught, although mostly in simplified formats. Takata's North American audience outside of the Japanese-American community in Hawaii was predominantly Caucasian. At the onset of World War II, anti-Japanese sentiment ran high, and a healing system or spiritual movement with a pronounced Japanese flavor would probably not have survived.

In addition to the simplification or removal of the Japanese techniques, Hawayo Takata told an altered form of the history of Reiki. Much like a fable or parable, this Reiki story was a teaching tool meant to impart necessary spiritual and moral lessons in addition to providing a pseudo-historical explanation of Reiki. Over the years, the history has been explored so that more factual data has been integrated into our current understanding of Reiki.

Takata's changes to Usui Reiki Ryōhō made it more palatable to Western practitioners and planted the seeds for Reiki to grow. Without Takata's ability to transmit the soul of the Reiki system through her dynamic teaching style and embellished historical narrative, Reiki may not have survived at all. Her passion and commitment to Reiki, as well as her adherence to the *gokai,* inspired students of all backgrounds to grow with Reiki.

Hawayo Takata continued to teach Reiki throughout Hawaii, and eventually on the mainland in the United States and Canada. She shared Reiki extensively and was for a time the only instructor outside of Japan. In the last years of her life, however, she began to train and initiate other teachers. Her travels led to the widespread practice of Reiki in a variety of communities worldwide.

One of the primary reasons that Takata-sensei may have changed the name she used for her training from Usui Reiki Ryōhō to Usui Shiki Ryōhō is that she was preparing for the eventual need to pass on her system. Takata seems to have believed that Reiki in Japan may have died out or gone underground, and she needed a plan to preserve it as she had known it and taught it. If Nishina's research is correct, Hawayo Takata only received the title of *shihan* from Hayashi. Since she was not a *dai shihan,** or senior teacher, she was not authorized to teach other *shihan*. Because Takata had been urged to begin training successors (see below), she would need to develop a means to do so without dishonoring her teacher and lineage. Just as Hayashi left the Usui Reiki Ryōhō Gakkai amicably to form his own institute with its own set of practices and protocols, Takata may have conceived of Usui Shiki Ryōhō so that she could train her own *shihan,* who would by then be known as Reiki Masters.

PROLIFERATION AND GLOBALIZATION OF REIKI

Although Hawayo Takata taught many classes across the globe, her students are responsible for the globalization of Reiki Ryōhō. Takata coached twenty-two students to the third degree, calling them Reiki Masters, just as she called herself. This group of students disseminated Reiki to global audiences one class at a time, and each of them adapted the system, either by default or by design, as the practice was spread. With a new generation of teachers, Reiki was shared with new students at an accelerated rate, eventually leading to the millions of practitioners worldwide today.

Takata's Twenty-Two

In 1976,[†] Takata-sensei began the process of training other Reiki Masters, or *shihan*. At that point, the Master training cost ten thousand dollars, which limited the number of candidates. Only those who were truly

---

*In 1930s Japan, the expression *dai shihan* was probably not used explicitly; even senior teachers probably only ever received the formal title of *shihan*. However, senior teachers would have been explicitly authorized to confer the status of *shihan-kaku* or *shihan* to other practitioners.

[†]In 1975, shortly after having her first heart attack, Takata trained her sister Kay Yamashita as a safeguard to ensure that someone else could transmit the system if she, Takata, passed away. The following year, Takata began to train others in earnest.

dedicated worked out a means of paying for the class. Hawayo Takata knew that her time was limited so she began to train those students who showed their dedication to Reiki. All in all, she trained twenty-two *shihan,* or Reiki Masters, between the years 1976 and 1980 (see page 76).

Takata was a dynamic teacher and she generally taught Reiki as an oral tradition. Students were not permitted to take notes or keep copies of the symbols in most instances. This caused confusion after Takata-sensei's death. When her *shihan* convened, they noted variations among the ways that their symbols were drawn. Takata also instructed her students—of all degrees of training—according to their needs, which sometimes meant that she adapted her teachings so that they would be best understood and appreciated by those in attendance.

When Hawayo Takata passed away, many of her twenty-two *shihan* met to decide how to continue the system of Reiki without her. Two organizations arose in response to confusion regarding Takata's chosen successor (or possible lack thereof). The first of these groups formed just prior to Takata's death; it was the American Reiki Association, which would later defect from Takata's teachings and become home to a form of Reiki called the Radiance Technique. The other group, which formed just after Hawayo Takata made her transition, is the Reiki Alliance. The alliance recognizes Takata-sensei's granddaughter Phyllis Furumoto as her successor. Today the Reiki Alliance continues to flourish, with members across the globe. To this day, Phyllis Furumoto teaches Reiki as her grandmother did.

Altering Takata's System

Takata's Masters continued to use the title Usui Shiki Ryōhō for the most part, until the Radiance Technique (called Real Reiki or Authentic Reiki at that point) broke away from the rest of the Reiki community. When it did so, it claimed to have the "complete" system of Reiki, consisting of seven levels taught exclusively to founder Barbara Weber Ray by Takata-sensei. This claim caused a rift among Reiki practitioners, and several of Takata's third degree students chose to practice and pass on Reiki independent of either Reiki organization.

SHIHAN, OR MASTERS, TRAINED
BY HAWAYO TAKATA

NAME	THIRD DEGREE	LIVED
Kay Yamashita	1975	?–?*
Virginia Samdahl	June 5, 1976	1918–1994
Ethel Lombardi	June 11, 1976	1922(?)–2009
John Harvey Gray	October 6, 1976	1917–2011
Iris Ishikuro	November 1976	?–1968
Harry Kuboi	April 18, 1977	1930–2013
Barbara McCullough	June 25, 1977	1924–2000
Dorothy Baba	July 10, 1977	1917–1985
Ursula Baylow	August 1978	1911–1996
Fran Brown	January 15, 1979	1924–2009
Phyllis Furumoto	April 1979	1948–
Barbara Weber Ray	September 1, 1979	1941–unknown
Barbara Brown	October 12, 1979	1915(?)–2000
Bethal Phaigh	October 12, 1979	1914–1986
Wanja Twan	October 12, 1979	?–
Beth Gray	October 18, 1979	1918–2008
George Araki	November 1, 1979	1932–2006
Paul David Mitchell	November 1, 1979	1946–
Shinobu Saito	May 1980	?–2015
Patricia Ewing	September 7, 1980	?–
Mary McFadyen	September 7, 1980	1931–2011
Rick Bockner	October 12, 1980	1948–

*As indicated by the question marks, some of the details about the dates of the lives and terms of the individuals listed above remain to be verified. The most detailed accounts of each of Takata's Masters can be found in *The History and System of Usui Shiki Reiki Ryoho* (148–180) by Robert N. Fueston. At the time of writing, only Phyllis Furumoto, Paul Mitchell, and Rick Bockner are still teaching.

In time, one of Takata's twenty-two *shihan* made a decision that would impact the rest of the Reiki world. Iris Ishikuro was initiated into Reiki by Hawayo Takata as the tenth Reiki Master; she taught both *shoden* and *okoden* together. Iris Ishikuro initiated only one other Reiki Master in her practice, a man named Arthur Robertson. Iris implored Arthur not to charge the ten-thousand-dollar fee for Reiki Master training. Robertson honored this wish and Reiki spread like wildfire. Arthur also updated Reiki by adding the kanji hand mudras, the Johrei symbols, and the Breathing Technique (Fire Dragon Breath and Contracting Technique) and called his method Raku Kei Reiki. This branch would serve as the foundation for many others, such as Terra Mai Reiki, Usui/Tibetan Reiki, and Karuna Reiki.

Today there are scores of different styles of Reiki, most of which can be traced to Hawayo Takata. Through the many stages of evolution in the last three and a half decades, Reiki has become infused with many outside influences, most of which are a result of the Western New Age and metaphysical movements. Ideas pertaining to the chakras,* auras, angels, ascended masters, crystal healing, shamanism, and color healing—as well as additional symbols—have been tacked onto Reiki's traditional methods as it is adapted by subsequent generations of Reiki teachers and practitioners.

REEMERGENCE OF TRADITIONAL REIKI PRACTICE IN JAPAN

Beginning in the 1980s and 1990s, word of Japanese lineages of Reiki untouched by the West had begun to emerge from Japan. Initially, there was very little hard data to support these claims, but Reiki practitioners from previously unknown lineages began to share their understanding of Reiki with several notable researchers. Over the last couple of

---

*According to Kurt Leland (*Rainbow Body*, 374), it appears that the first time the chakra system was linked to Reiki Ryōhō was in 1985, in Bodo Baginski and Shalila Sharamon's *Reiki—Universale Lebensenergie*, later published in English in 1988 as *Reiki: Universal Life Energy*.

decades, the history of Reiki Ryōhō has been rewritten, and our catalog of traditional practices and methods has grown considerably.

Before outlining the efforts of some of the more notable people who have contributed to our new understanding of the origins of Usui Reiki Ryōhō, it would be appropriate to dispel a few persistent myths that have arisen during the last twenty years. With the increasing popularity of research into the original teachings of Usui Mikao, the number of false sources has also been on the rise. Unfortunately, several public figures have made claims about their teachings, asserting that their sources were Usui's or Hayashi's original students.

These pseudo-historical claims have attempted to revise Reiki history to suit the agendas of some teachers. Ample charisma and an understanding of Japanese culture can lend authenticity to even the wildest of claims, which has made Reiki-related research more difficult in recent years. When such revisionists are pressed about their sources, however, none of those sources can be verified. Be cautious about stories of Tendai nuns, Tibetan sutras, or other ideas that conflict with an accurate understanding of Reiki history.

Frank Arjava Petter's Research

Arguably the most influential figure in Reiki research, Frank Arjava Petter was the first person to offer a translation of the memorial stone erected by the students of Usui Mikao in 1927. In the 1990s, Arjava lived in Japan for many years and was the first person to offer Takata-style Reiki training in all three degrees, which attracted many students from around Japan to his seminars. His experience with the language and culture of Japan has afforded him many opportunities to connect with entirely Japanese styles of Reiki.

Arjava-sensei has written numerous books on Reiki, each disclosing new research into its origins and methods. His work has included contact with the former president of the Usui Reiki Ryōhō Gakkai, Ms. Koyama, as well as several other people trained in lineages that trace back to the *gakkai.* His works have included the translations of many important articles, booklets, and instruction manuals, and as a result Western audiences are able to read them for the first time. He has collected various articles, certificates, rare photographs, and many other primary sources that allow us to see how Reiki was practiced and taught decades ago.

The earliest insights into the original Japanese Reiki Techniques surfaced through Arjava-sensei's efforts. In the late 1990s, he began to travel to the West to offer training in these techniques. There are now many practitioners and organizations across the globe that have reincorporated the Japanese Reiki Techniques into their curricula. (For more information on these tools, please see chapters 8 and 18.) Arjava later befriended the Yamaguchi family during his work with Reiki. He would eventually be appointed the vice chairperson of the Jikiden Reiki Kenkyukai. Today, he continues to travel worldwide, offering seminars in Jikiden Reiki and pursuing his passion for Reiki history.

Doi Hiroshi and the Usui Reiki Ryōhō Gakkai

Doi Hiroshi is an influential figure in the dissemination of accurate, updated historical information on the practice of Usui Reiki Ryōhō, which is due to his past affiliations with the society founded by Usui-sensei himself. Doi first learned about Reiki in the 1980s, and he later attended the first and second degree seminars in the 1990s with Mieko Mitsui, a student of Barbara Weber Ray.[39] Doi was led to believe that the original forms of Usui Reiki Ryōhō had died out, a belief that was also prevalent in the United States at that point. However, several years later, Doi met a woman who had been a member of the Usui Reiki Ryōhō Gakkai for more than forty years.[40] She introduced him to the *gakkai* and Doi was soon inducted into the association and initiated by then-president Koyama-sensei.

Initially with the blessings of the *gakkai*, Doi was permitted to share his newfound understanding of Reiki and an accurate version of the history of Reiki in Japan. Because the *gakkai* does not accept foreigners into its ranks and because joining, even as a Japanese person, is extremely difficult, Doi synthesized the styles of Reiki that he had learned into Gendai Reiki Hō, or Modern Reiki Method. Through his work with the Gendai Reiki seminars, Doi has been able to create a system of Reiki that honors the best practices of both Eastern and Western styles of Reiki and provides important historical information to the world. Doi's system of Reiki and his historical research are available in his recently revised book, *A Modern Reiki Method for Healing.*

Doi-sensei was among the very first traditionally trained Japanese practitioners to begin sharing original teachings with Western audiences. In 1999, he traveled to Canada for the Usui Reiki Ryōhō International Conference in order to present Gendai Reiki Hō training. He continued to participate in the next three conferences. Doi's teachings have helped practitioners worldwide bridge Western and Eastern methodologies to create a combined tool kit for a variety of circumstances.

Yamaguchi Chiyoko

Yamaguchi Chiyoko was born in Kyoto on December 18, 1921, with the maiden name of Iwamoto. Coming from a large family of seven children, Chiyoko was sent to live with her uncle Sugano Wasaburo, who had no children of his own. She moved to Tezukayama, near Osaka, while in the second grade. Not long thereafter, Chiyoko and one of her brothers moved to Ishikawa with her relatives, the Ushio family. It was while living here that she first learned the word *Reiki.*[41]

Sugano Wasaburo first studied Reiki Ryōhō with Hayashi in Osaka in the late 1920s. He soon introduced the practice to his family in Ishikawa. In 1935, Hayashi-sensei traveled to Daishōji, Ishikawa, to teach *shoden* and *okuden* as a five-day seminar. Within three years' time, a satellite branch of the Hayashi Reiki Kenkyukai was established in Daishōji. That same year, on March 13, 1938, Chiyoko began a five-day course consisting of *shoden* and *okuden* together, taught by Hayashi himself.[42] Approximately two years later, Chiyoko was taught how to perform *reiju.*[43]

Chiyoko married Yamaguchi Shosuke in 1942, and she continued to use Reiki pervasively. Her children were raised with Reiki and received both treatment and *reiju* from their mother. Reiki was a folk art in families like the Yamaguchis', and it replaced the need for conventional medicine when allopathic care was less widely available. The Yamaguchi family continued their practice of Reiki throughout times of war and poverty. Over time, Chiyoko and her son Tadao began to study other healing systems as a means of better understanding Reiki.[44]

Chiyoko-sensei began teaching Reiki to others in 1997, originally without a strict curriculum, distinct degrees of *shoden* and *okuden,* or certificates.[45] As she gained more students, her classes became more structured, especially with the assistance of her son Tadao. Together they founded the Jikiden Reiki Kenkyukai, an organization that aims to preserve Hayashi's teachings through their Reiki seminars. Jikiden (直傳) means "by direct transmission," implying that the courses are the same as was traditionally taught by Hayashi-sensei. Nishina, himself a *dai shihan* in the Jikiden Reiki Kenkyukai, writes, "To clarify what and how Hayashi taught Reiki, Chiyoko and Tadao Yamaguchi visited their relatives to collect notes, photographs and their [relatives'] recollections. Their efforts brought about a complete recovery of Hayashi's teaching. Therefore the contents of Jikiden Reiki are based not only on Chiyoko Yamaguchi's memory, but also on the information kept by her relatives."[46]

In 2003, Chiyoko passed away peacefully. Her son continues to teach Reiki and has grown the institute since her death. Thanks to the diligent efforts of the Yamaguchi family, the teachings of Hayashi Chūjirō have been maintained in a largely unaltered form and given to the world today. Tens of thousands of practitioners have been trained in these original methods of Japanese-style Reiki. The Jikiden Reiki Kenkyukai tirelessly researches and disseminates new findings that pertain to Reiki's history, and they have been able to publish many important resources. Teachers of Jikiden Reiki undergo rigorous training in order to deliver Reiki training according to the same standards of practice that Hayashi himself once implemented.

REIKI TODAY

Reiki has enjoyed exponential proliferation since Takata-sensei made her transition. Authentic and unaltered lineages from Japan have been rediscovered, as have new documents and photos revealing the history of Reiki. The many varieties of Reiki extant in today's world are a testament to the versatility and perseverance of the spirit of Reiki.

The history of Usui Reiki Ryōhō is still an incomplete picture. As a result of the passage of time, it may be impossible to fill in all the gaps. Many researchers and teachers are working hard to replace spurious claims and misinformation with facts about Reiki that are supported by evidence, Usui Mikao's work and vision, and the spread of Usui's teachings. In the next few years snippets of new information that may help clarify the roots of Reiki will no doubt surface.

Reiki is an ever-changing phenomenon. While the energy of Reiki remains the same, the practice continues to reform and adapt as practitioners and teachers grow in number. As a global Reiki community, it is our duty to assimilate current research into our perspectives of Reiki in order to ensure its accuracy and authenticity for future generations. Although sifting through the sands of time is often a painstaking process, we are challenged to maintain a beginner's mind so that we continuously see the system with new eyes. As researchers unearth new information, our beliefs surrounding Reiki Ryōhō may be challenged. In spite of this, we must remember that the real teacher is Reiki itself. One's practice is seldom made more effective by memorizing dates and names; it is enhanced by diligent, heartfelt work.

If something should come to light that is at odds with your understanding of Reiki or its history, always remember to turn to Reiki itself for the answers. Although hands-on healing or *gasshō* meditation can't tell you when or where something happened, it can help resolve the materialistic need to "own" that information. It may be enough to know that, as Reiki practitioners, teachers, and enthusiasts, we are living history.

Scientific evidence is mounting in support of the therapeutic value of Reiki, and studies will continue to be conducted in order to further explore this. Likewise, in order to advance spiritually, seekers the world over are drawing inspiration from the roots of Reiki and the spirit of its founder. Reiki is truly a blessing, and it will likely continue to support and catalyze the evolution of our world, one *kokoro* at a time.

4

THE REIKI PRECEPTS

AT THE HEART OF THE REIKI TRADITION is a short document scribed by Usui-sensei that we briefly mentioned in chapter 1 and that we will elaborate on here. Known colloquially in Japan as the *gokai,* which means "five admonitions," the simple instructions contained in this document are guidelines for attaining inner peace and complete balance of body, mind, and spirit. Although there are many practitioners today who push the five precepts to the back of their minds once class is over, these principles really are the heart and soul of Reiki practice and should be a central focal point of contemplation at all times.

Usui-sensei traveled the world, worked in politics, and underwent a silent retreat at a Zen monastery in Kyoto. He sought out many different tools and walked many paths before teaching Reiki Ryōhō. The *gokai* are a distillation of the many studies of Usui-sensei. Knowing that he spent much of his life dedicated to higher learning, we would do well to heed his suggestion of applying ourselves to these principles. They are the core of his teachings for a reason, for they reflect the thread of universal truth that Usui found among his diverse experiences. The Usui Reiki Ryōhō Gakkai, Hayashi Reiki Kenkyukai, and Jikiden Reiki Kenkyukai have continued the tradition of reciting the Reiki Principles at each meeting, before initiation, and sometimes even before treatment.

Again, in Japanese, the five precepts are usually called *gokai,* although a few other terms for them also exist. In the handbook used by the *gakkai,* the precepts are introduced as *kyōgi* (教義), which translates as "principle," "creed," or "doctrine." Dr. Hayashi uses the term *ikun* (遺訓) on his hand-brushed scroll of the precepts. *Ikun* means "legacy" or "dying wishes," implying that these teachings are the heart of Usui's practice. An alternative title for the precepts was introduced by Reiki instructor and author of *O-Sensei: A View of Mikao Usui,* Dave King, in his Usui-dō system; he proposes that the text is actually referred to as the *gainen* (概念), meaning "concept." There is, however, no evidence to support this claim, nor do any of the practicing Reiki organizations in Japan make use of the term *gainen* with relation to the precepts.

ORIGINS

Over the last couple decades there has been a fair amount of speculation about the origins of the *gokai.* After initial contact with Japanese practitioners of traditional Usui Reiki Ryōhō, Western Reiki practitioners believed the *gokai* to have been inspired by the Meiji emperor of the late nineteenth century. Much of the reason for this is that Usui-sensei used the poetry of Emperor Meiji as a teaching tool; 125 of these poems chosen by Usui are still included in the handbook of the Usui Reiki Ryōhō Gakkai.

The poems of Emperor Meiji were helpful tools for teaching morality, diligence, and other ideals; the *gokai* are a later innovation. Given that Usui was crafting a system of spiritual development for laypeople, he strived to provide clear guidelines that were simple and practical, not to mention effective. He probably culled from many resources, both spiritual and secular, to arrive at the final two drafts that exist today.

Frans Stiene is a Reiki Master/Teacher, cofounder of the International House of Reiki and the Shibumi International Reiki Association, and a critically acclaimed Reiki author. He and other teachers have noted the similarity between the Five Principles and the Six Paramitas of Buddhism.[1] The paramitas are called the six perfections, and they represent the pinnacle, or perfection, of six different virtues. It is known that Usui attended grade school at a Pure Land (Jōdo Shū) Buddhist temple, and that he practiced in a Zen monastery later in life, just before his awakening to Reiki. Therefore, it is quite possible that the paramitas may have served as a source of inspiration for him, despite the fact that less tenuous connections can be made to other probable texts.

It is likely that the provenance of the *gokai* comes from a text called *Kenzen no Genri* (健全の原理), or Principles of Health/Soundness.[2] The author of this Japanese text, Dr. Suzuki Bizan, appears to have been an adherent to (or at the very least influenced by) the New Thought movement, a philosophy that began in the United States in the nineteenth century and influenced many of the *shinshūkyō* of Japan. New Thought teaches that the Divine is in all things, spirit is the totality of real things, the true nature of humanity is divine, sickness begins in the mind, and correct thinking has a healing effect. You'll notice a correlation between these principles and those espoused by belief systems and spiritual practices in Japan, especially Shinto and Reiki Ryōhō. *Kenzen no Genri* was published in 1914, approximately eight years before Usui-sensei ever climbed Mount Kurama. In it, Dr. Suzuki writes:

> A Path to Soundness
> Today only
> Be not angry
> Be not fearful
> With honesty
> Perform diligently your duty
> Be kind to others
>
> BIZAN[3]*

---

*In his book (*Reiki: The Transmigration of a Japanese Spiritual Heaing Practice,* 322), Reiki Master and researcher Jojan Jonker provides the original Japanese text of this poem as "今日だけは, 怒らず, 恐れず, 正直に, 職務励み, 人に親切" (*kyō dake wa, ikarazu, osorezu, shōjiki ni, shokumu wo hagemi, hito ni shinsetsu*).

These principles and those of Usui are startlingly similar; however, not much is known about Dr. Suzuki today, so we can only conjecture what influence his writings may have had on Usui Mikao. No matter what the precise origins of the *gokai* are, research has repeatedly indicated that the truths they contain comprise the very heart and soul of Usui Reiki Ryōhō and its many offshoots. Usui himself advises us to recite these phrases as if they are affirmations, so that they can guide us to improving heart-mind and body.

THE PRECEPTS IN JAPANESE

To better understand the *gokai* in any language, one can look at the source material in Japanese. Two versions exist; one is allegedly brushed in Usui's own hand, whereas the other is carved into his memorial stone, erected by his students. One can only understand these versions fully after learning to appreciate the culture out of which they have come. An examination of Japanese psychology, spirituality, and orthography reveals the meaning hidden within these simple statements. It is also true that they contain a deeper meaning than one might initially surmise.

Both Japanese versions of the text stress the importance of practicing the precepts just for today. The vocabulary in each differs slightly, although the overall message remains the same. We will examine the translations below, with some explanation of what the deeper message of the chosen kanji truly means.

Brushed Version

招福の秘法　　萬病の靈薬
今日丈けは怒るな
心配すな　　感謝して
業をはげめ　　人に親切に
朝夕合掌して心に念じ口に唱へよ
心身改善臼井靈氣癒法
初代臼井甕男

Shō fuku no hihō   manbyō no rei yaku
Kyō dake wa   ikaru na
shinpaisu na kanshashite
gyō wo hageme   hito ni shinsetsu ni
asa yū gasshō shite kokoro ni nenji kuchi ni tona e yo
shin shin kaizen Usui Reiki Ryōhō
choso Usui Mikao

The secret method of inviting good fortune
The spiritual medicine of all illness
Today only   Anger not
Worry not   Be grateful
Be diligent in your work   Be kind to people
Morning and evening do *gasshō,* hold these in your heart, and chant the principles
Heart-mind and body Improvement: Usui Reiki Ryōhō

FOUNDER, USUI MIKAO[4]

Memorial Stone Version

一二日ク今日怒ル勿レ
二二日ク憂フル勿レ
三二日ク感謝セヨ
四二日ク業ヲ励メ
五二日ク人ニ親切ナレ

ichi ni iwaku kyō dake was ikaru nakare
ni ni iwaku ureuru nakare
san ni iwaku kanshaseyo
shi ni iwaku gyō o hageme
go ni iwaku hito ni shinsetsu ni[5]

First we say: today only do not anger
Second we say: do not fear (or do not be anxious)

Third we say: be grateful

Fourth we say: work with diligence

Fifth we say: be kind to people[6]

Kotodama

The reason that reciting the principles in their original language persists today in countries around the globe can be found hidden in a cultural perspective from the birthplace of Reiki. Known as *kotodama* or *kototama,* it is the belief that words inherently have power. In kanji, *kotodama* is written as 言靈; the second character should look very familiar to students of Reiki! Literally, the expression means "word spirit/soul" and refers to the living force that animates words.

Kotodama implies that sounds are sacred. In many spiritual traditions around the world, Creation stories are described as beginning with a word or song. This primal reverence of the creative power of sound is the same belief that empowers students of *kotodama* to harness the mysteries of language for esoteric workings. Much like the Shinto belief in kami—the gods, devas, or souls of natural forces, beings, and objects—the soul of the word is the force responsible for the life within written and spoken language.

The complexity of the Japanese language, especially in its written form, can be daunting to foreign students. However, the characters themselves have such charm and beauty that one can't help but sense something mystical empowering them. *Kotodama* is put into motion as these words are spoken, thus invoking the spirit or consciousness of their sounds into one's life.

Understanding the idea of *kotodama* is important for comprehending why the Reiki *gokai* are meant to be recited aloud. The ideals are more than just affirmations to help program the mind; they are like prayers or mantras to invite the "spiritual medicine of all illness" to guide and direct one's consciousness. It is likely that the exact wording of the *gokai* was chosen to access specific *kotodama,* which means that only by speaking these words aloud can one truly reap the benefits of the Reiki Principles.

The practice of *kotodama* may have been popularized by one of the leaders of the Oomoto Kyō (a new Japanese religion originating from Shinto), Deguchi Onisaburō (1871–1948), and by the founder of aikido, Ueshiba Morihei. Deguchi was a spiritual pioneer and political activist; Ueshiba was his student. Ueshiba engineered aikido to embody the practice of *kotodama,* believing the martial art to be the best way of using it. Today, one can find a number of books on the subject of *kotodama* in a variety of languages. Similar animistic beliefs about words and sacred sounds are practically universal. We can thus effectively apply the *kotodama* principle to our practice of the *gokai* in any language.

Although the soul of the Reiki Principles may be best felt in their native tongue, they are ideals that transcend the barriers of language and culture. The *gokai* are spiritual directives that guide us toward the realization of inner peace: *anshin ritsumei.* Although we are specifically asked to recite the *gokai,* Usui-sensei looked for those practitioners who sincerely lived by and embodied the principles to be candidates for *shinpiden.* By chanting the principles, especially in their original forms, we invoke their power to transform our lives. We can follow Usui's example and use the Reiki Ideals as guideposts along our individual paths to awakening.

COMMON ENGLISH RENDERINGS

When Hawayo Takata taught Reiki to students (for approximately four decades), she generally subscribed to an oral tradition for transmitting the teachings. Because of this, and because of her dynamic and adaptable teaching style, the Reiki Ideals were often presented with different wording for different audiences. She had the wisdom to make the inherently Japanese system of Reiki Ryōhō available and comprehensible to Western minds. An additional reason that many versions of the *gokai* exist today is that her students initially carried on the oral tradition that Takata-sensei established, sometimes reaching back decades into their memory banks in order to pass on the Usui System as they had learned it.

Below you will find a few different presentations of the Reiki Principles in English. Most of them trace back to Hawayo Takata and her twenty-two *shinpiden* or Reiki Master students. As these principles were shared from teacher to student, the order changed slightly, as well as their superficial flavor and vocabulary. Despite this, the underlying sentiment remains the same. If the Japanese principles feel too foreign, cumbersome, or uncomfortable to you, try using one of the following for your daily practice instead.

From the "Blue Book" (a pamphlet called *The Usui System of Natural Healing*) of the Reiki Alliance by Paul David Mitchell, one of Takata's twenty-two teachers:

> Just for today do not worry.
> Just for today do not anger.
> Honor your parents, teachers, and elders.
> Earn your living honestly.
> Show gratitude to every living thing.[7]

From Fran Brown, another of Takata's twenty-two teachers:

> Just for today: Do not ANGER
> Just for today: Do not WORRY
> Just for today: COUNT YOUR BLESSINGS, honour your parents, teachers, and neighbors. Eat food with gratitude.
> Just for today: LIVE HONESTLY.
> Just for today: BE KIND TO ALL LIVING THINGS.[8]

From the biography of Virginia Samdahl, the first of Takata's twenty-two teachers:

> Today I will count my many blessings. I will give thanks and be faithful.
> Today, just for today I will not worry.

Just for today I will not be angry.
Today I will do my work honestly.
Today I will be kind to my neighbor and every living thing.[9]

From Mary Hodwitz, who studied with Takata in June 1979:

Just for today, not to anger.
Just for today, not to worry.
Count your blessings; give thanks for food, for water, for parents,
for friends, for fresh air.
Earn your living honestly.
Be kind to everything that has life.[10]

From Judy-Carol Stewart, a member of the Reiki Alliance:

Just for today thou shall not anger.
Just for today thou shall not worry.
We should count our blessings and show our gratitude.
Do an honest day's job, earn an honest living.
Be kind to anything that has life.[11]

From Beth Gray, one of Takata's twenty-two teachers:

Just for today—
Do not worry, Accept
Do not anger, Accept
Count your blesings
Do an honest day's work
Be kind to all living things[12]

From author and teacher Paula Horan:

Just for today, I will live the attitude of gratitude.
Just for today, I will not worry.

Just for today, I will not anger.
Just for today, I will do my work honestly.
Just for today, I will show love and respect for every living thing.[13]

From a handout made by Takata and given to students in 1975:

Thou shall not anger
Thou shall not worry
Thou shall count your blessings
Thou shall revere your parents, teachers, and friends
Thou shall earn an honest living
Thou shall be kind to all living things*[14]

The *gokai* reinterpreted (by me) as affirmations:

Just for today, I release my anger.
Just for today, I release my worries.
Just for today, I am grateful.
Just for today, I devote myself to my work.
Just for today, I am kind.

An alternate translation by Reiki author Frans Stiene:

The esoteric teachings to invite blessings
The spiritual medicine of having strayed from universal truth:
Today only
Do not anger
Do not worry
Be grateful
Practice this diligently
Be kind to yourself and others

---

*This version expresses the third principle as two separate admonitions; it is also one of the few extant versions without the reference to "today" or "just for today."

Perform Gasshō in the morning and evening
Be mindful about this in your heart/mind
Chant with your mouth
Improve your heart/mind and body
Usui's teachings (dharma) to cure and heal one's True Self[15]

EXPLORING THE PRECEPTS IN DEPTH

The Reiki *gokai* seem simple at first glance. However, the principles themselves are the backbone of the Usui System of Natural Healing; they are the guidelines of one's spiritual practice. The *gokai* are tools to enhance one's skill set, and their simplicity underscores their sincerity, for spiritual truth is always simple.

Usui called the *gokai* "the secret method of inviting good fortune" and "the spiritual medicine of all illness." The grandeur of these titles should not be taken lightly. Reiki Ryōhō founder Usui Mikao truly must have believed in the mental/emotional and spiritual benefit of reciting the *gokai* so much that he thought they would precipitate even physical healing. For this reason, each of the Five Principles will be illuminated in greater detail below.

Today Only: 今日丈けは

Nearly all adaptations of the Reiki Principles begin with some reference to the present moment. "Just for today," "today only," and even simply "today" precede the five admonitions as a reminder that the work we must do is in the here and now. Only in the present moment can we truly make any progress at all.

Looking at the Japanese text of the *gokai* gives us a clue to the importance of the phrase *kyō dake wa*. It is the only place in the *gokai* where the particle *wa* (は) is found. In the Japanese language, particles serve as identifiers for different parts of speech; they may indicate which words in the sentence are the subject or object, among many other grammatical functions. *Wa* is generally considered to mark the topic of a sentence. While the particle *wa* does not necessarily indicate the subject of a sentence or passage, it does help center the focus on the word or phrase it modifies. Since none of the official admonitions in the *gokai* contain the topic-marking *wa*, it stands to reason that Usui-sensei used this particle to highlight the importance of "just for today." Thus, *kyō dake wa* points to the central message of the entire *gokai*; if we do nothing else, we can live in the here and now and still accomplish what Usui admonishes.

In order for the following guidelines to be actionable, it is necessary to take things one day at a time. Usui-sensei surely would have deemed it unreasonable to ask his students to cease being angry once and for all. Similarly, it is nearly impossible to just flip a switch and never worry again. The primary reason that the *gokai* are framed by *kyō dake wa* is because only by taking things one day at a time can we commit to the directives laid out in the precepts.

Each new morning brings rebirth, and the Reiki Principles point our heart toward this simple truth. Perhaps you were angered yesterday; maybe your heart was full of anxiety. And yet the practice of Reiki is unhindered by your past and your future because it is a practical method for achieving wholeness *right now*. When you feel uncomfortable or when conflicting emotions bubble up, just take a breath and remind yourself, "Just for today . . ."

Kyō dake wa (Just for today) has become a favorite mantra of mine. When I start to get ahead of myself or worry about an impending deadline, I can center myself simply and clearly by reciting this short phrase. The more I do it, the easier it becomes, and that is one of the blessings of Reiki Ryōhō. Reiki is a spiritual method for achieving wholeness by "improving heart-mind and body" (*shin shin kaizen Usui Reiki Ryōhō*). By practicing the *gokai* in real time, the results hasten; it's exactly the same as training your physical body except that you're flexing your mental muscles with the *gokai*.

The Reiki Ideals begin with "just for today" to remind us to make time for our practice *today*. That means every day. When you don't think you have time for it—when you are feeling the most overwhelmed—that's when you need it the most. Pause and reflect. Give yourself

Reiki by placing your hands wherever they are most comfortable. If you're out in public, you can surreptitiously lay them flat on your thighs or on some other inconspicuous place on your body. Reiki is so easy that it doesn't require complicated props or sequences in order to flow. You just have to make enough space in your mind (and heart) to receive it.

"Today only" applies to every principle in Usui's "secret method." Today you can release your anger. Today you can resist worrisome thoughts. Today you can turn toward gratitude. Today you can really commit to your work. And today you can practice kindness and compassion. Small steps make the practice easy to digest; no one expects you to give away all your belongings, radically change your diet, and move into a monastery overnight after your initiation into Reiki. If that was the goal, there wouldn't be a point of practicing at all.

Although not officially a separate admonition, *kyō dake wa* deserves equal attention. A beautiful thing gradually takes place as we live by the "just for today" principle. We start to really live out the principles automatically, as if by some mysterious guidance. Living for today opens the door to our intuition and invites indescribable joy.

Anger Not: 怒るな

The first principle is often rendered "do not anger" or "do not get angry" in English. In Japanese, the character for *anger* is comprised of the radical for *slave* (奴) and for *heart-mind* (心).[16] When we become angry, we are a slave to the fiery emotion that overtakes our heart and mind. Rage is a powerful emotion and often stems from unmet desires, which are themselves forms of attachment. Anger is a grasping onto what cannot be; it shares similar roots with disappointment and envy.

For some of us, anger is our natural state. It is a learned way of life because it seems to absolve us of the responsibility of controlling our circumstances. Anger enables us to displace whatever feelings of shame, guilt, or disappoint we harbor; it is a means of misdirection. We have all met people who are perpetually angry, and there is nothing we can do to please them because they cannot please themselves.

The first principle falls beside "today only" in both surviving Japanese texts of the *gokai.* This implies that the first principle is an extension or refinement of living in the now. When we are angry, we are attached. Again, this feeling typically results from a past action or outcome that did not fulfill expectations. When we give in to anger, we are living in the past. There is no growth to be had in the past because we cannot change it.

By focusing on living in the now, we are gifted with the beautiful opportunity to embrace life as it is in the present moment. Reiki Master Beth Gray reminds us of this in her restatement of the ideals when she writes, "Just for today do not anger—Accept." Acceptance is not the same as resignation. It doesn't mean that you've given up; it only means that you have given up an attachment to what isn't working. By not allowing yourself to be engulfed in rage, you can maintain a mind that is clear enough to course-correct. Clear thinking provides the best chance to navigate through difficult situations.

Releasing your anger as it arises in the moment can most easily be achieved through conscious breathing. When you begin to feel the heat of anger rising, remind yourself, *kyō dake wa ikaru na* (today only, anger not), and shift your awareness toward your breath. Breathe fully and deeply. Let the pace of your inhales and exhales slow down. Your body will naturally relax and your mind will follow. This is one of the keys to putting your mind to work for you, instead of being its slave.

The first principle isn't just saying "don't stay angry." It's ultimately asking you not to get angry at all. Any healthy spiritual practice is geared toward retraining the mind. "Just for today, don't get angry" means you are training your mind not to go there; rage doesn't serve your growth. It makes things hazy and it clouds your judgment. When you submit to your anger, you aren't capable of making healthy decisions. For this reason, Usui-sensei's reminder is to focus on being right here, right now . . .

Although anger is harmful when misused, it can sometimes provide the necessary impetus to change. When we experience fear, grief, and shame, anger is typically a sign that we are ready to make a change. A common motif in several Buddhist traditions is that of "wrathful deities." These beings have fearsome faces and are often surrounded by flames. Wrathful gods share rank with many bodhisattvas and other enlightened beings. They have mastered their anger and are channeling it into positive change; wrathful deities lead us into enlightenment.

When anger faces you, be sure to put it to work for you. Let it be the wake-up call that says, "Change is necessary." Train yourself to respond to anger with forgiveness. Replace rage with peace by focusing on the breath, and you will be well on your way to spiritual awakening.

Worry Not: 心配すな

Up to a certain point in my life I could have written the definitive guide for how to worry. I found a way to worry about everything, practically all the time. My life was a tangled mass of deadlines and emails and schedules and stress. It didn't matter if it was during my academic years or my professional years; changing the setting didn't change my mental patterns.

Worry was my natural state. It was easiest to fret about the future because it was my default setting; I'd built a habit of replaying my worries incessantly. However, the more diligently I practiced Reiki, the easier it became to relax. Letting go of worry is rarely easy, but the trick is to remember the beginning of the *gokai*: just for today . . .

The word for worry is made up of two kanji: 心 and 配. The first is *kokoro*, in this case pronounced *shin*, and it means "heart." The latter character is read as *hai* or *pai* and translates as "distribute." To worry is to literally distribute your heart's wholeness. When you give in to anxious feelings, your vitality and peace disintegrate and drift away. Worry gives away your power; it is sometimes called a prayer for chaos.

By learning to live in the now you can prevent the stress-related effects of worry. Anxiety is (usually) a milder form of fear, as indicated by the inscription on Usui's memorial stone. On the inscription, the second principle can be read as "sorrow" or "fear." Fear stems from impending circumstances, which steer us away from the present moment. These worries generally come from an inability to relax into the unknown. An easy antidote is to remember how the *gokai* begin, and it's for this reason I have made *kyō dake wa* my personal mantra for many years now. Each time I invoke its *kotodama,* anxiety melts away a little faster.

If we are to be able to offer healing to anyone, we must learn to take care of ourselves first. One of the most effective ways to do so is to adopt healthier thoughts and emotions. Worry can seem innocuous on the surface, but this harmlessness is a false front. A worrisome heart has holes eaten through it. Stress compounds and affects your immune system, digestive system, and even your metabolism. Learn to live in the now and let tomorrow come in its own time.

Like the first principle, the second is a further refinement of "just for today." A worried mind is focused on future events and their unknowable outcomes. Thus to truly experience today only, you have to relinquish the future as much as the past. You cannot know peace without letting go of attachment, and that is one of the lessons Usui hid within the *gokai.* As you train your heart-mind to dwell in the ever-present now, emotions like anger and fear fall by the wayside.

When you practice Reiki Ryōhō you are opening yourself to be a vessel for divine energy. You learn to accept this in a passive way. In a similar fashion you can learn to let go of worry by merely accepting each circumstance as it arrives, without judgment or hurry. You don't need to become powerless by absolving yourself of the authority to change, but you also don't need to make yourself sick with anxiety over what can't be changed.

One of my favourite ways to support this precept is with hands-on Reiki. When you feel stressed, place your hands wherever worry becomes palpable; for me this is usually around my chest (heart) and solar plexus. Focus on your breathing and let the Reiki flow. Worry can dissipate quite rapidly this way.

Practice Gratitude: 感謝して

In kanji, *gratitude* is created from the word for feeling, *kan* or 感, and the word for thanks, *sha* or 謝. The expression *kanshashite* comes from the verb *kanshasuru,* which means literally "to make" or "to do" gratitude (or appreciation). The first character in the word for gratitude combines the root, which means "unison," with the character for heart-mind, the *kokoro.*[17] In other words, it means uniting the heart and the mind. Gratitude is the state that brings the mental and emotional fields into perfect unison for the sole purpose of being appreciative.

Gratitude is one of the most fundamental spiritual practices. It can transform your mood, your health, and your life circumstances. It is a practice that naturally directs your focus into the present moment, because it is hard to be grateful for something that is no longer here or that which hasn't happened yet. Being thankful opens doors to higher consciousness by elevating your mood and counteracting stress.

Feeling thankful and showing your appreciation are two halves of the same coin. The inception of a grateful heart is a receptive act. Expressing it is the key to balancing the equation; when you send that feeling outward and share it with others, you empty yourself enough to make room for new reasons to find thanks.

Because *kanshashite* and *kanshaseyo* (from the brushed version and memorial stone, respectively) can be translated as "show appreciation," Takata-sensei often used this principle as a reminder to honor the important people in your life. Asian cultures, particularly the Japanese culture, have a long-standing tradition of honor and respect. Respecting your elders, teachers, parents, and those who have helped you along your life path is a quintessential part of the social psyche. In the West this practice has diminished in recent generations; as Reiki practitioners we would do well to take Takata's expansion of this principle to heart.

One way to show appreciation in your Reiki practice is to honor your Reiki lineage. Although the family trees of most modern-day practitioners' lineages are quite complex, we can always trace our Reiki heritage back to Usui Mikao, the founder. Most of us in the West also owe our practice to Hayashi Chūjirō and the *shihan* (instructors) he taught such as Hawayo Takata and Jikiden Reiki founder Yamaguchi Chiyoko. Displaying a photo of the *shihan* is a helpful way of offering gratitude to them.

Practicing gratitude makes the world a happier, healthier, and more abundant place. The *gokai* contain the admonition to show your gratitude because it is one of the simplest shortcuts to spiritual growth and healing that you could ever hope to use. Each day as you awaken or drift off to sleep, you can merely place your Reiki-charged hands anywhere on your body and revel in your gratitude for having the gift of Reiki. Try to conjure a short list of all the experiences for which you have thanks. Before you know it, your life becomes more aligned with your divine purpose.

The Reiki Principles teach you to live in the present moment, which means being thankful for what you have rather than fretting about what is missing. Reiki Ryōhō as a spiritual practice intends to return the human condition to its original experience of utter perfection. You are already complete just as you are, and as you awaken to your true self, you will recognize your indelible, inseparable connection to the Divine Source.

Be Diligent in Your Work: 業をはげめ

On the surface level, the fourth principle in the *gokai* seems to be pointing toward honesty and integrity in your work. As it has been handed down by many teachers as "do an honest day's work," this principle is often the one that many spiritual practitioners struggle with. It can be hard to align your heart to this principle until you understand its deeper message, which is more than merely to work hard.

We live in a world that no longer rewards dedicated work the way it once did. This is largely due to the lack of authenticity in the workplace today. We train for specialized careers in order to make money rather than to fulfill our heart's most intimate dreams. Earning an honest day's work, however, isn't necessarily about the money. This precept is a gentle reminder that we must be honest with ourselves about what we are here on Earth to accomplish.

In Japanese, this admonition uses the character 業 (*gyō*), which variously means "profession," "deed," "training," "practice," "skill," or "karma." Its influence stretches far beyond our concept of a job. *Gyō* is derived from an ancient ideograph depicting a complex instrument, implying the great amount of skill and training necessary for mastery.[18] The fourth principle is really nudging us to make a commitment to our practice; that is the essence of the translations offered as "be diligent in your work."

Applying ourself diligently toward spiritual healing and growth chips away at the ego and reveals the authentic self beneath. The work we do can take many forms, such as meditation, journaling, counseling, or perhaps hands-on Reiki. In addition to working on our own skills, "work hard" means to commit to self-care. We can't exhaust ourselves in the process of evolution without ever pausing to take care of our needs. It is vital to set aside time for relaxation and fun in order to have equilibrium in our lives.

The fourth principle links us again to the injunction of "just for today." It is the principle of mindfulness made manifest. As we work, either for personal development or in a professional setting, there is a certain magic that takes place when we use our whole awareness to do the task at hand. We replace trying with doing; we allow things to unfold instead of forcing them. The secret is the involvement of the heart.

Being present in our work recalls the Taoist concept of *wu wei,* meaning "doing without doing." We open our hearts and still the mind. In this space when we work we are not complicating our tasks with mental gymnastics; rather, we are simply being present with the task. There is a stillness in *wu wei* that belies the great amount of work really being achieved. Through the concept of heart-centered focus in all that we do, we can more readily tackle the important tasks of our lives.

Gyō also implies a sense of duty, which is so strongly instilled in the Japanese group consciousness. We must uphold our duty, or obligations, to ourselves, our teachers (such as Usui-sensei), and our society.

This does not mean living the ideal life as portrayed in the normative stereotypes of our day. Fulfilling your *gyō* involves living the best life for you, not for someone else. By reaching for your potential you are honoring all those who have helped, trained, or believed in you.

Striving for personal excellence also makes you an example for everyone you meet and work with. By aligning your outer world with your inner truth, you can inspire and empower those around you to do the same.

The penultimate precept asks you to show up for your practice every day. In relation to your Reiki practice, this means taking time for Reiki every day. Give yourself Reiki, share it with your loved ones, send it to your goals, bless your food with it—just use it. You cannot grow in your Reiki if you do not hone it. Empty yourself of the attachment to outcome and just do it, mindfully and with sincerity. The rest will happen on its own.

Show Kindness: 人に親切に

When Hawayo Takata shared this precept with her students she widened its scope from the original Japanese text. The expression is literally rendered as "be kind to people," but Takata emphasized that this principle is not limited to human beings. We can show kindness to our neighbors, our loved ones, strangers, and everything that has life.

The final admonition helps us cultivate a lifestyle of compassion. We can put compassion into action through the mind-set of showing kindness. Kindness helps us connect with individuals around us on a human level. We can show kindness in many ways, from smiling at the register when we check out at a store to being kinder, more patient drivers. The opportunities for putting this precept into action are endless, as are all of the possibilities that are inherent in Reiki.

When we cultivate compassion, we develop empathy for others. We are invested in the suffering of the world, not because we cannot tear ourselves away from its horrors, but because we believe that there is a way through and a way out. When we direct this compassion to those around us, human and otherwise, we generate merit, which equates to good karma. One of the most fundamental laws of the universe is that we reap what we sow; therefore, each act of kindness paves the way for a better life for us all.

It is important to recognize that any kindness that does not begin with onself is insincere. The only lifestyle of compassion that is complete is one that includes self-compassion. "Show kindness" asks you to take time for you. If you are ill, exhausted, overworked, or just having an off day, be gentle with yourself. Examine your thoughts and you will start to recognize when you are and aren't being kind to yourself. How often do you think things such as "I'm terrible at this" or "I hate myself for doing that"? These are unkind sentiments that you can overcome with diligence.

Yamaguchi Chiyoko believed that one way of embodying the fifth principle involved more than being kind to others. She also advised, "Give them or teach them Reiki!"[19] Sharing Reiki with the world helps you fulfill your duty, or *gyō*, to Usui-sensei; it also helps you practice kindness by offering a means of healing others.

Kindness is a way of life. Find compassion in your heart by releasing your judgments and your expectations so that kindness can flow easily. One of the easiest ways to help someone heal is to just show up with your whole self; be really, authentically, wholly present with him or her. That level of intimate kindness may be even more effective than laying on of hands during a Reiki treatment. When you are living this principle, the force of unconditional love supersedes any other programming that you might have, and it will guide you through your life.

❖ Personalized Precepts

Now that you have seen the Reiki precepts presented in a variety of formats, take some time to evaluate how you can benefit from them. Which one(s) will be the easiest for you to put into action? Which will be the most challenging? The *gokai* shouldn't necessarily be easy, despite their plain and straightforward mandates. Growth requires challenge, and the *gokai* challenge Reiki practitioners to aspire toward the example left by Usui Mikao.

Take some time in an undisturbed place to ponder the five admonitions. With some paper and pencil at the ready, write down the numbers 1 through 5. Think about each of the Five Principles and put them into your own words. Refer back to the translations provided of the original texts in Japanese, as well as the versions left to us by Takata's legacy. Take your time and polish your choice of words until they really shine.

Be sure to have fun with this. Will you phrase each one similarly? Does *just for today* get its own line, or will you repeat it with each admonition? You can state the principles as affirmations or use a commandment-like voice. Restating the *gokai* in your own words encourages you to take ownership of them. It is an invitation to bring them into your *kokoro* (heart-mind) and make them a daily practice. Being able to personalize these guidelines also promotes a deeper comprehension and retention of their meaning. Most of all, it proves that you are willing to go one step deeper with Reiki as a spiritual practice.

MAKING THE *GOKAI* A DAILY PRACTICE

There are many practitioners around the world who receive a copy of the precepts in their first degree class and pay scant attention to them. The principles are overlooked by many Reiki lovers because their interest lies in the hands-on healing applications that Reiki offers. Although Reiki practice does open the doorway to physical healing through laying on of hands, the lasting cures come from mental and spiritual healing.

Usui Mikao writes: "First the mind should be healed, and secondly the physical body be made healthy as to walk on the right path of humanity. If the mind is healthy, conforming to a path of integrity, then the body becomes sturdy of its own accord."[20] Our founder is explaining that the principal aspect of healing is not physical; spiritual practice retrains the mind and brings the emotions into balance. This is why the *gokai* are at the heart of Reiki Ryōhō.

Remember that Reiki began as Usui-sensei condensed his many years of spiritual study into a system that could bring even laypeople to an experience of imperturbable peace. The goal of Usui Reiki Ryōhō is inner peace: *anshin ritsumei*. As practitioners, when we apply the principles conscientiously, they serve as tools to transform our minds. Naturally, the body follows the mind and the spirit, and healing takes place at every level.

Reiki was not unknown before the time of Usui Mikao, which is why he titled his method differently, thereby specifying it as 心身改善臼井靈氣癒法 or Shin Shin Kaizen Usui Reiki Ryōhō.

Rather than simply calling his teachings Usui's Reiki Healing Method, Usui-sensei specified that it was the method for "improving mind and body." Even the order in which these two aspects are listed shows that the mind (and therefore the heart, as they are not separated in Japanese psychology or spirituality) has greater importance in healing than the physical aspect of reality. Modern science is uncovering an enormous relationship between these two parts of ourselves, and mind-body medicine is a rapidly growing area of study.

Although with the miracle of *reiju* we are granted the healing power so abundantly praised in Reiki, the most sacred aspect of the tradition consists of the *gokai*. Therefore, we can honor Usui's teachings and take our lives into our own hands by merely choosing to live by the principles. Each day we can remind ourselves of their importance by reciting them or meditating on them; this simple act can change your life.

Usui's Instructions

At the end of the calligraphy that records the *gokai,* Usui-sensei instructs Reiki practitioners how to use the precepts. We are told "morning and evening do *gasshō,* hold these in your heart, and chant the principles." He is imploring us to make the *gokai* a daily practice so that we can internalize and embody their spirit in all that we do, not just during the time we mindfully practice Reiki healing.

The instructions begin with the kanji for morning and evening. If we take just a few moments twice each day to reflect on the Reiki Principles, then we frame all of our activities by their influence. The *gokai* are meant to be tools for navigating through life toward the attainment of spiritual realization and *anshin ritsumei.*

One Reiki researcher, Dave King, suggests an alternate meaning behind these characters.[21] By treating them as a compound word in lieu of two separate times of day, the message conveys the idea of practicing the *gokai* throughout the day, literally "from morning to night."* Although this is not a historically sound way to interpret and pronounce

---

*As a compound word, these kanji are pronounced *chōseki* instead of *asa yū.*

this section of the document, I think it does capture the deeper meaning of what Usui-sensei expects from us. Instead of simply chanting the principles when we awaken and before retiring, Usui Mikao expected dedicated Reiki students to *live* the principles, as if each moment they were in a prayerful state (as suggested by doing *gasshō*).

Before reciting the *gokai* aloud, the instructions ask us to hold the concepts in our heart, or *kokoro.* This directive uses the Japanese term 念じ, or *nenji.* This word can mean both "remembrance" and "silent prayer." Reiki *shihan* and author Frans Stiene writes, "In essence this means deeply bearing the precepts in your heart/mind. This means to become the precepts, to embody them in your heart."[22] When you hold them in your *kokoro,* your heart *and* your mind, the precepts are planted in fertile ground. Making a daily practice of it waters and tends to these spiritual seeds so that they may blossom.

Usui explicitly asks us to hold our hands in *gasshō,* a mudra similar to the conventional prayer position, and to chant the *gokai* out loud: *"Gasshō shite . . . kuchi ni tona e yo."* One of the reasons for speaking these words is to invoke their *kotodama.* If we use Usui's sacred words each day, it becomes possible to receive the essence of his original teachings.

❈ Meditations on the Precepts

The Five Principles of Reiki serve as a road map for personal development. They can be applied in a myriad of ways, so feel encouraged to use your meditation to further guide you here. In addition to chanting the principles each morning and evening, meditating on the precepts (*kokoro ni nenji*) is also recommended by Usui-sensei. Reflecting on them, as a whole or in part, helps you live and breathe the *gokai.*

You can meditate on the entire text or focus on a single precept at a time. I would recommend finding the wording that is the most meaningful to you. Although the Japanese text has the strongest feeling behind it, being able to relate to what you are contemplating is important. When you've settled on the version of the *gokai* that you would like to use, choose the principle with which you'd like to work. Start with a single precept per day and stick with it throughout the day.

Spend a few moments in silent reflection, with your hands together in *gasshō*. Invite the blessings of Reiki to flow through and around you. Empty yourself of expectation and attachment as you do so. Now, focus on your chosen principle. Let's use "just for today do not worry" as an example. You can connect to it in your native language or in Japanese (*kyō dake wa shinpaisu na*). Recite the principle silently as you reflect upon its deeper meaning.

As thoughts arise, don't worry about trying to suppress them. Just let them come and go freely. There is no need to chase them away; merely observe them. It is likely that with some patience, your inner resistance to the meaning of the precept will arise. For example, if you're meditating on releasing worry, your own worries and anxieties may show up. Consciously acknowledge them and send them into the light of Reiki. Whenever you are ready to end your meditation, thank the guidance of Usui Mikao and Reiki itself. If you would like, recite the Five Principles to signal the end of your meditation and return your awareness to your surroundings.

With practice you can cycle through each of the principles in a given week, or you can reflect on all five at once. If you would like to have a different meditation for each day of the week, you can reflect on the double title that Usui uses (*shō fuku no hihō, manbyō no rei yaku*, "the secret method of inviting good fortune, the spiritual medicine of all illness") on the first day, "today only" on the second, and one of the Five Principles on each of the remaining days, thus giving you seven unique themes, one for each day of the week. Making a daily practice of reflecting on the principles deepens your connection to the origins of Reiki, thereby augmenting your ability to channel Reiki for any application. Try this out and see how it changes your practice.

❸ *Gokai Sansho*

This meditation, called *gokai sansho* or 五戒三唱, means "three recitations of *gokai*." The *gokai* are sometimes used in Japanese branches of Reiki as a means of preparing both the inner and outer space before initiations, meditations, and even treatment. Chanting the text in Japanese invokes the *kotodama* as it was originally programmed into the *gokai*. This simple exercise can be used at the start and end of your day, as well as any time you would like to create a sacred space for your Reiki practice.

To start, place your hands together in *gasshō.* Focus your attention where your middle fingers meet, and breathe deeply and rhythmically. Clear your mind and prepare to speak the Reiki Ideals. Traditionally, we are taught the version of the text in brush form rather than the inscription from the memorial stone, but try the one that you feel the most drawn to. Speak in a clear voice and an even pace, with your eyes closed if you have the text memorized.

When you have finished, spend a moment in silent gratitude before concluding your exercise. You may compare the energy, or *kotodama,* of the Japanese text to your favorite versions of the Reiki precepts in your native language. More than likely, you'll feel the Japanese text to have a stronger influence on the energy of your space. Take a mental inventory of how you feel before and after *gokai sansho* as a means of checking its efficacy.

Once you've learned how to say the principles, they can be used for a quick rebalancing wherever you are. Recite them when you awaken to set the tone for the day. Speak them aloud before or during a Reiki treatment to help clear the energy and strengthen your connection to Reiki itself. (For help with pronunciation, please see appendix B, which contains a phonetic guide to reciting the principles. There are a multitude of recordings available online, too.)

In the next chapter we will look more closely at the human body and its energy field, for a proper understanding of this is important for a full comprehension of how Reiki works to enhance healing.

5

HOW REIKI HEALS

ANCIENT HEALERS UNDERSTOOD that the whole world and everything in it is comprised of vibrating fields of energy, including the human body with its own energy field. Contrary to the perspective that the paradigm of Western medicine posits today—that physical ailments are ailments of the body only—more esoteric healing modalities such as Reiki posit that disease (*dis-ease*) first occurs in our energy field before permeating the denser levels that we know as the human body. Whenever we are spiritually or emotionally out of balance or alignment is when we are most vulnerable to falling prey to any manner of illness—mental, physical, emotional, and/or spiritual. This chapter will explore how Reiki works specifically on the human body and its energy field to restore health and discusses what other areas of life it can aid.

EVERYTHING IS ENERGY

Everything in the known universe is comprised of tiny components that sometimes behave like matter, wherein they are called particles, and sometimes behave like energy, making them waves. Each of these tiny wave-particles is in constant motion, meaning that every solid object we encounter isn't quite as dense as it seems. All matter vibrates at rates unseen to the human eye. The moving particles also generate their own energy fields, which provide a veritable sea of frequencies through which we swim each day.

Conventional medicine generally assumes a mechanistic perspective of the human being. We are inert matter, and the energy fields produced by the body are merely a side effect. Complementary and alternative therapies like Reiki work within a vitalistic worldview; they view the body as responding to a vital energy or life force. Energy fields produced by the body are as important as physical tissue because of the information that they contain and relay.

This concept is still being explored by modern science. Indeed, science and medicine are working together in order to explain the effects of energy medicine. Reiki has become well documented by a growing body of literature. Slowly and steadily the scientific community is demonstrating that biofield therapies are the future of medicine. Reiki may one day be as mainstream as a regular checkup with your family physician or a visit to the dentist.

THE HUMAN ENERGY FIELD

Surrounding the human body is a measurable field of electromagnetic energy that's referred to as a biofield, biomagnetic sheath, or L-field (as in "lifefield") by many scientists today. Each cell in a person's makeup contributes to the overall composition of his or her energetic body, although the heart and brain are the primary drivers of this phenomenon. Studies have shown that this envelope of electromagnetic energy contains information about the health and well-being of the individual it surrounds. Disease, attitude, and biological cycles can be detected by analyzing this energy field.

From a spiritual perspective, the nature of the human energy field has been known for millennia, and it is most often referred to as the aura. Traditionally, the aura has been depicted as a circular or ovoid field of light or energy surrounding and penetrating the physical body. It is composed of various layers of energy fields, each becoming denser as one travels from the outermost reach toward the center. The densest field of them all is the physical body itself; it is under the influence of each of the finer, more rarefied fields around it.

The various layers of the aura—including the spiritual, karmic or causal, emotional, mental, and supraphysical or etheric—respond to life in unique ways. Your attitude, thoughts, environment, activities, and diet can influence your nonphysical anatomy, which in turn affects your physical body. Many illnesses manifest first at the energetic level before making their way into physicality; this is why Usui Reiki Ryōhō seeks to heal the mind first and then the body.

Within the aura are a number of other nonphysical "organs." These subtle structures include the chakras, nadis, and meridians. Chakras are like vortices of energy located at major points of intersection between the physical and subtle anatomy. Traditional views count seven major chakras, with scores—possibly hundreds—of minor centers. Nadis and meridians are energy pathways. Meridians are mostly relegated to the physical body, whereas most nadis are situated within the aura. (Detailed descriptions of the aura and the chakras may be found in appendix A.)

The *Tanden*

Information about the chakras and aura is not native to the practice of Reiki. *Chakra* is a Sanskrit word that reflects the philosophy of Vedic cultures as relayed down through time. When Usui Mikao taught Reiki to his thousands of students, there was no mention of Reiki's effect on these aspects of our subtle anatomy. Usui-sensei instead used Japanese concepts such as the *tanden* when describing how Reiki works.

The *tanden* (丹田) are three energy points in the human body. Sometimes conflated with the chakras, *tanden* have similar functions but are culturally distinct from any of the seven major chakras described elsewhere. The three *tanden* are the upper, lower, and middle. The lower of the three is the one of greatest concern to Reiki Ryōhō. It is also referred to as the *hara,* as well as *dantian* in Chinese. Located very close the second chakra, the lower *tanden* is approximately two finger-widths below the navel.

In Japanese and Chinese martial arts, this *tanden* is one of the main foci for cultivating personal energy. Ki can be stored and concentrated here through meditation, movement, and breathwork. In the practice of Reiki, the energy of Reiki flows down through the top of one's head and to its seat at the lower *tanden.* Several Japanese Reiki Techniques and meditations make use of the *tanden;* we will explore in chapter 12.

Reiki's Effects on the Human Energy Field

Despite the lack of historical veracity for claims about the effects of Reiki on the human energy field, the experience of countless practitioners demonstrates that Reiki is effective for healing at the auric level. It also can ameliorate budding problems in any of the chakras. Because Reiki is focused first and foremost on healing the spiritual and mental-emotional aspects of our being, it exerts its influence over the subtle anatomy before stepping down its vibration into physical reality.

When we become vessels for channeling Reiki energy during a *reiju* or attunement, the subtle bodies and other spiritual parts of our anatomy are adjusted or rewired for Reiki. Reiki flows in through the top of the head at the crown chakra and continues downward to the lower *tanden* or *hara,* in the abdomen. From there, Reiki flows up into the heart and along the arms and into the palms. Usui Mikao taught that Reiki naturally flows through the palms, the feet, the eyes, and the breath. This means that we can use any of these for administering Reiki. It courses through the entire human energy field of the practitioner, so that each time a practitioner gives Reiki, he or she is also receiving it.

The Mechanism of Reiki in Healing

When we lay hands on our recipients (or direct our gaze or our breath onto them), Reiki enters the energy field and physical body near where the hands are placed. From there it gradually saturates that area and spreads out. Targeting the source of a healing opportunity—such as the site of injury or a point of origin of disease—will increase the efficacy of the Reiki treatment because it can most directly influence the area in question. This is why Japanese traditions encourage practitioners to

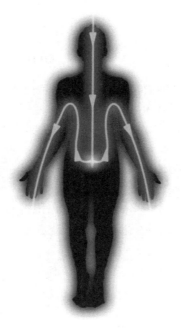

Reiki first flows to the practitioner's lower *tanden*
before traveling through the hands during treatment.

follow their intuition and heed the cues of *byōsen*. For the same reason, Takata developed the Foundation Treatment to ensure that all areas would receive Reiki. (The Foundation Treatment is a complete treatment and as such it targets all the major parts of the body. It will be discussed in greater detail later in the book.)

Reiki flows through the practitioner via a passive mechanism; it is actually the body (or mind or spirit) of the recipient that draws the energy of Reiki on an as-needed basis. Because of this, no conscious effort or direction is required by the practioner. Instead, Reiki will flow as it is needed. There may even be occasions when it does not seem to be flowing at all. Such instances may arise from the recipient not needing the support that Reiki offers.

Reiki works by stirring up disharmony so that it can be released or resolved. This can translate to a variety of different movements or processes. Reiki may work on the subtle bodies by releasing negative energies from the aura. It can sweep away foreign thoughtforms or entities or sever energetic cords. In the chakras, Reiki may improve the flow of energy, remove blockages, correct imbalances, or reconfigure the chakra vortex itself if it is marked by leaks, tears, or stretched energetic structures. Analogous benefits can be found among the nadis and meridians; they may be freed of blockages so that normal ki flow is restored.

Reiki seeks out any areas that conflict with our divine heritage, which means that it can offer healing on any and all levels of our existence. As practitioners, when we place our Reiki hands on ourselves or another individual, Reiki flows to where there is disharmony in order to restore order. It is especially effective at seeking out stored toxins, both physical and subtle. As Reiki is flowing, practitioners often report physical sensations in their hands or bodies, a phenomenon that Usui called *byōsen.*

Byōsen is discussed in greater detail in the chapter 7, but, in short, it's the state of energetic resonance between practitioner and recipient that allows for the Reiki practitioner to sense or palpate how Reiki is working. Varying degrees of intensity in the *byōsen* indicate different states of imbalance. This can indicate how long to treat a given area as well as where to apply the symbols after receiving the training in *okuden.*

No matter how you visualize Reiki working, its mission is to support awakening to our highest spiritual truth. In order to achieve enlightenment or awakening (*anshin ritsumei*), we must have order restored to our bodies and minds. Reiki helps us achieve this balance by inundating us with compassion and unconditional love—a frequency that reminds us of our true nature.

A RETURN TO HOMEOSTASIS

Reiki can be used in meditation, in contemplation, or as a conventional hands-on treatment to support the homeostatic mechanisms of the human being. Homeostasis is the tendency toward a stable equilibrium among all the distinct, interdependent elements of a system.

In biological processes, homeostasis is evidenced by the natural order of physiological well-being. When injury or illness offsets this delicate balance, the body sets certain events in motion to return to equilibrium. Examples are the efforts of the immune system or the repair of broken bones.

Reiki supports the homeostatic mechanisms not only at the physical level but also at the psychological and spiritual levels. Reiki energy flows to the root of a given condition, which can mean that physical pain may be resolved by healing emotional turmoil first. Sometimes, when we treat a specific target area, Reiki flows to another part of the body where the condition originates. It can similarly flow to a mental, emotional, or spiritual condition or energy in some other part of our being in order to ameliorate what is being treated. Since Reiki is an intelligent force, the practitioner does not need to know or diagnose the origin of the issue for Reiki to be effective.

Finding Balance: Mind before the Body

As previously stated, the founder of Reiki Ryōhō initially designed the system to act primarily as a program for personal development and spiritual growth. By healing the mind and nurturing the soul, Reiki naturally extends its influence to the denser levels of our embodiment. It is as if Reiki heals from the inside out, first reaching into the core of any issue or concern. Healing the causal pattern underlying physical or emotional stress clears the entire plethora of concerns. The reason that Reiki is so effective is because it removes the cause as well as the symptom instead of treating only the symptom.

In leading us to homeostasis, Reiki works to bring the body, mind, and spirit back into balance. No single part of ourselves can be treated independently because it does not exist in a vacuum. Reiki joyously and lovingly helps us integrate mind-body balance as well as resolve any conflict between the spiritual and secular aspects of our life. The primary tool for achieving this balance is the *gokai;* this is followed and supported by the art of *tenohira* or "hand healing."

The Healing Reaction

Often during the course of a treatment protocol, the client's symptoms may appear to worsen. Perhaps this manifests in the form of diarrhea, pain, fever, or general malaise. Because Reiki's primary action is to help detoxify the body and spirit, clients may undergo a healing reaction or healing crisis. The body is responding to the energy of Reiki and is beginning to eliminate the toxins, pathogens, and harmful energies that are contributing to illness.

Hawayo Takata would admonish her students to continue treating despite an appearance that the condition had taken a turn for the worse. Fever, vomiting, sweating, diarrhea, and urination are all means by which the physical body expels harmful substances. When we're treating chronic conditions, the healing reaction is likely to last several days; remember that if we didn't get sick overnight, it isn't likely that we'll get well overnight. When a healing reaction occurs it is imperative to continue treating with Reiki.

As Reiki practitioners it is also imperative to remember that we are not permitted to diagnose or cure any condition. When our clients begin to experience the healing reaction we must encourage them to seek the opinion of their medical professional of choice. We can also offer insight into other times when we have seen the healing crisis work its magic during Reiki treatments. Although it's important to avoid diagnosing symptoms, we are able to illustrate the likely effects of the reaction by sharing our own experiences.

The healing reaction can vary from mild to severe, and it is always contingent upon the severity of the conditions being treated. As you offer Reiki to your client, you can check in energetically with the underlying cause by sensing the *byōsen* in his or her body. Continue to treat the cause of the illness, rather than switching your focus only to the new symptoms manifested by the healing crisis.

Many practitioners undergo a similar healing reaction after their initiations into Reiki. These are typically very mild, and they can be ameliorated by daily self-treatments. Be gentle with yourself, drink more water, and eat healthy foods. With diligent practice, Reiki will help you achieve balance on all levels.

WHAT CAN REIKI TREAT?

At the most basic level, Reiki is often viewed as relaxing and effective for managing pain. Many practitioners market their Reiki practice to mainstream audiences by billing it as a Japanese technique for stress reduction. Although this isn't incorrect, Reiki offers so many more benefits to the human being. Below we will take a closer look at what and how Reiki Ryōhō treats at each level of one's being.

Physical Benefits of Reiki

The *shoden* level of Reiki is primarily focused on the physical level of healing. Most Reiki teachers encourage new practitioners to use self-treatment every day and to give as many treatments as feasible to others to practice at the *shoden* level. It is not uncommon for diligent and hopeful practitioners to experience their first Reiki miracle within the first few weeks of their initiation. Relief from pain, the mysterious disappearance of cuts, burns or bruises, and many other miraculous transformations can and often do take place.

Common effects of Reiki treatment include pain management, first-aid applications, improved digestion, better sleep, relief from acute and chronic illness, higher energy levels, and a stronger immune system. Scientific studies have documented a number of physiological benefits of Reiki, such as reduced impact from stress and a shorter recovery time from injury or illness. Reiki supports every biological process, and because it treats at the root level, Reiki can bring lasting results. (It is, however, important to remember that chronic conditions require several treatments in order to achieve a return to wholeness.)

In order to describe how Reiki works on biological systems, it's important to understand that cells are influenced by electromagnetic fields. Healthy tissues and organs have constituent cells that are working together to emit a unified, coherent field of energy. Yet when disease or injury affects the behavior of these cells, their energy fields lose the coherency that is a characteristic of health.

Many types of healers, including Reiki practitioners, have been shown to emit very strong fields of energy from their hands. The energy of these fields has been measured as being more than one thousand times greater than the energy that the rest of the body emits.[1] Since the tissues of the body act as a liquid crystal system, the energies emitted by the practitioner can be distributed throughout the body and energy field of the recipient. The crystallinity of biological tissue transmits messages and energies very well, which explains how Reiki can travel to the origin of an issue, even when it is "unknown."

It's also important to realize that the energy of Reiki flows from the universe through you before ever reaching the energy field and body of your client. This means that you never use your own energy when healing another. It also means that, as a practitioner, each time you treat another person, you are also being healed. Reiki offers its abundance of blessings to all, and it never needs replenishing.

More than anything, you should remember that regular practice will enhance your Reiki treatments. To deepen and augment your healing abilities, practice Reiki daily and connect to the precepts. Although there are measurable, scientifically viable mechanisms that can be observed in Reiki, the mystery of the system begins with a spiritual experience: the initiation. Reiki helps heal the physical body because it heals the soul, and it carries this healing down through the successively denser fields of energy that comprise the whole being.

Mental-Emotional Benefits of Reiki

Psychological well-being is the most tangible benefit of Reiki. After a Reiki treatment, one feels refreshed, alert, relaxed, and peaceful. The mind is clear and ready to work in harmony with the rest of one's being. Out of balance emotions are reined in so that they can be quietly and lovingly processed or released. Reiki combats all manners of stress, and it can help heal the mental or emotional echo left by trauma.

Because the most effective way to administer Reiki is through physical contact, Reiki practitioners give a rare gift to their clients, that of mindful, compassionate touch, which is largely nonexistent in today's world. Especially outside the family group, seldom is touch ever exchanged without expectation. In Reiki, touch is not transactional; it is never given with the expectation of receiving something in return. Loving contact can help the body release hormones that elevate the mood and improve overall well-being.

Reiki as a healing art is based on *tenohira* or *teate,* the Japanese form of "hand healing." In any culture, touch plays a role in intimacy, fulfillment, and emotional well-being. Physical contact recalls the soothing touch of the archetypal mother, who reaches to soothe her child's every wound. Because of this, the corporeal relationship between practitioner and recipient can fill the need for human contact. This in turn soothes emotional wounds by lifting depression, alleviating anxiety, and calming turbulent emotional states such as fear and anger.

Usui Reiki Ryōhō is a form of mind training. This is evidenced in the Five Principles themselves—and more so in the instructions for implementing them as inscribed by Usui. Our founder knew and taught that healing the mind naturally heals the body, so he left the precepts as a tool for doing just that. When we practice Reiki mindfully, we are not only offering healing energy to our clients, we are also engaged in meditative practice. Being present and sincerely compassionate during hands-on Reiki opens the door to our own mental-emotional healing.

Practicing Reiki can take many forms. Apart from the obvious hand placements, Reiki can be used in quiet reflection or meditation as a means of healing the psyche. Because it automatically offers a push toward achieving equilibrium, Reiki restores mental and emotional balance. Connecting to Reiki during contemplation or meditation is a shortcut to harmony. Reiki enhances the outcome of meditative endeavors, thereby enabling an individual to take their psychological health into their own hands.

Try meditating with Reiki in different ways. Contemplating the Reiki Principles can be a simple exercise to obtain psychological benefits from Reiki Ryōhō. You can do this in focused stillness or while walking through your favorite scenery. This powerful way of performing moving meditations calms the mind and allows your spirit to shine through and lead the way to wholeness.

In the second degree or *okuden* class, students are introduced to a specific symbol for healing emotional and mental conditions. Hands-on Reiki as it is taught at the first degree and the *gokai* are adequate tools for addressing many psychological conditions as they relate to overall wellness. However, students are encouraged to take their practice deeper by participating in and enjoying the next class (*okuden*) in order to learn tools and techniques for addressing these concerns directly.

Spiritual Benefits of Reiki

Given that Reiki is literally "spirit energy" (see chapter 1 for a discussion of kanji), it naturally stands to reason that its primary effects are directed at the spiritual level of your existence. Every part of your body, each thought in your heart-mind, and every event you experience are results of your spiritual makeup. For each and every moment of the day, there is a part of your spiritual blueprint being read and translated into your reality.

Reiki functions to heal by enabling the true self to become visible. The more you devote yourself to practicing Reiki, the more in tune you become with the spiritual fabric of the universe. Reiki is fundamentally spiritual because our true nature is inseparable from the Divine. Reiki is nonreligious, but it is sacred. The experience of Reiki can provide a feeling of communion with the entire cosmos. The practice of Reiki Ryōhō equips you with the tools to empty yourself of attachment and expectation in order to be filled with the limitlessness of unconditional love.

Reiki clears away the spiritual cause of disease and disharmony. Opening to the infinite flow of Reiki can heal a person's perception of lack and scarcity just as easily as it can relieve pain or mental anguish. It is a call from our holy origins, which we can answer merely by accepting it. Since Reiki doesn't come *from* you, at least not the earthly you, it can bring tidings of your divine birth in the mind of God. Hawayo Takata often called Reiki "God power" in order to convey the intensity of its effects.

The practice of Reiki heals not only our disconnection from spirit but also our karmic patterns. By practicing Reiki we never take on the karma of illness or injury from our clients; we also do not prevent karmic lessons from being learned. Reiki helps fulfill our spiritual contracts by healing the root cause of conflict, whether it's physical, emotional, or causal. This means that Reiki will help the recipient integrate the lesson inherent in any situation so that the symptoms may be released once and for all.

When Usui Mikao had his awakening on Mount Kurama, his aim was not to produce a method of physical healing. He collected the pearls of wisdom from his many years of study and diligent practice and wrapped them up in the newly born system of Usui Reiki Ryōhō. His experience of enlightenment was so profound that he was inspired to make it available to us all. Because of his commitment to bringing *anshin ritsumei* to the world at large, Reiki was shared for many generations by his students. Usui Mikao left us the tools we need for spiritual growth and self-realization, and they are hidden in plain sight among the elements of the Usui System of Natural Healing.

REIKI AND OTHER HEALING PRACTICES

Reiki Ryōhō does not have to be practiced in isolation. It supports the application of various methods of restoring balance, including conventional allopathic medicine. Other holistic and complementary modalities may also be enhanced by using them in tandem with Reiki. Since there is no such thing as "too much Reiki," nor is there ever any contraindication related to its use, Reiki may be safely integrated into wellness routines amidst a plethora of other therapies.

Bodyworkers and practitioners of other touch-based therapies can use Reiki in conjunction with any other technique. Reiki seamlessly helps chiropractors, craniosacral therapists, massage therapists, Rolfers, reflexologists, and those healing professionals who employ osteopathic manipulation. Practitioners can disclose their Reiki training to clients or they may just surrender to whatever is best for the highest good of whoever is on the table. Sometimes Reiki will flow, and sometimes it won't, as the client's body will accept it only as needed.

When practicing other energy therapies, it may be necessary to make the conscious distinction between what is and isn't Reiki. Not only is this delineation helpful in maintaining the treatment protocols of each system, but it also ensures the integrity of Reiki as it's perceived by the recipients of healing. If bodyworkers do not inform their clients that they are combining methods or switching between systems, clients may become confused about what they do and don't like about Reiki or other therapies. Although this doesn't directly change how Reiki flows, it can certainly lead to conflation and misinformation in the community.

Therapeutic Touch, Integrated Energy Therapy, Healing Touch, Quantum Touch, Jin Shin Jyutsu, and other energy modalities can all be supported by Reiki. Similarly, homeopathic remedies, flower essences, and gemstone elixirs can be augmented with Reiki. In these instances, Reiki can be infused into the remedies themselves, and it can be administered to clients as they use the remedies. Crystal therapy, acupuncture, and virtually every other complementary and alternative treatment method can be infused with the blessings of Reiki in one form or another.

Because Reiki supports relaxation, it puts clients at ease. By releasing stress and entering a state of focused peace, clients are able to get the most out of any and every modality being administered. Around the world, health care practitioners of many types are learning how to add Reiki to their practice. Conventional doctors, osteopaths, nurses, psychotherapists, counselors, social workers, and many others involved in wellness are enhancing their practices with Reiki. When necessary, Reiki can be used discreetly, even without touch, as the need arises.

Reiki is an excellent tool to integrate into any holistic practice, for it deepens and prolongs the effects of healing techniques. Using Reiki in conjunction with other healing tools can be a rich and rewarding experience for practitioners and clients alike. Since Reiki Ryōhō benefits the practitioner, Reiki healers typically feel energized after sessions, even when they are applying other healing modalities, too. In this way Reiki is a multidimensional tool that can lead one into wholeness through many avenues.

THINKING OUTSIDE THE BOX

Reiki is not limited to healing only conditions of the body, mind, and spirit of individual human beings. Recent innovations in Reiki have seen it effectively applied to restore the health and well-being of plants and animals, as well as for promoting the peace and harmony of groups, organizations, and ecosystems. Reiki is the universal, cosmic energy of unconditional love, which knows no limitations or exceptions. In light of this, Reiki can be applied to virtually every aspect of life to support healthy, spiritually sound outcomes.

Reiki can be used to empower food and medicine. Place your hands over your comestibles prior to eating and drinking them to infuse them with Reiki energy. Reiki supports physiological health through nutrition, and it offers blessings of gratitude to each individual in the supply chain responsible for bringing your food and beverage from its origins to your table. Many people report that food and water taste different after being charged with Reiki.

Send Reiki to your goals by writing them on a piece of paper or a note card. Hold it in your hands and visualize Reiki flowing to the target situation. Remember to write your goal in an affirmative statement in the present tense. There's no need to work out the finer details; leave that to Reiki and to Source. In the second degree you will learn how to enhance and hasten this process by using the Reiki symbols.

Bless and empower your favorite crystals and gemstones with Reiki. Although Reiki is not an effective substitute for a thorough cleansing or clearing, it helps realign stones to their original blueprints much in the way it works with us. Reiki can also supercharge your gems for better results. Usui and Hayashi performed *reiju* on clear quartz crystals to provide continuous healing for clients who lived far away from practitioners; experiment with your own collection of crystals to see how Reiki interacts with them.

Charge candles and incense with Reiki and light them with a specific intention in mind. They will broadcast your intention alongside the Reiki to assist in the achievement of your goals and provide environmental equilibrium. You can also use Reiki to cleanse the energy of a room by chanting the *gokai,* as described in the last chapter.

Empower correspondence, gifts, and messages with Reiki so that the recipients may accept the Reiki in tandem with the letter or present. This makes a loving, gentle way to offer support for your loved ones on all levels.

These are just a few ideas for using Reiki to promote healing beyond the practice of the laying on of hands. No matter how you use it, know that it will work for the best outcome possible. Reiki offers no judgment, doesn't interfere with anyone's karma or destiny, and can cause no harm. Again, there is no such thing as too much Reiki, nor are there any contraindications to its use, so empower every aspect of your life with it. Reiki is adaptable, spiritually guided, and effective on all levels; it lends itself to any creative use you can imagine!

6

CONNECTING TO REIKI

THERE IS NO EXACT RITUAL OR PROTOCOL REQUIRED to connect to Reiki once we have received our first *reiju*. Initiation is the only prerequisite for implementing Reiki. For a practitioner of Usui Reiki Ryōhō, no conscious direction of the Reiki flow is needed to ensure its efficacy. To have a successful treatment, we just need to step out of the way and allow Reiki to take over. This does not mean our conscious mind is superseded by Reiki consciousness; rather, it means that we give permission for Reiki to flow where it is most needed by the recipient, whether that is to ourself or to another person.

LET GO, AND LET REIKI FLOW!

When we first become Reiki practitioners it's common to wonder if what we're doing is really working. The secret to effective Reiki treatments is to get out of our own way; learn to surrender and relax into it. There is no need to visualize the flow of energy or to picture the healing process taking place. Reiki is the driver during treatment, and both giver and receiver are going along for the ride.

Although it isn't necessary to undergo a complex procedure for beginning a treatment, it can be helpful to cultivate your own method of connecting. Creating a personal rite or technique helps you, the practitioner, approach Reiki with a consistent attitude, and it helps separate the time during treatment from ordinary consciousness.

This personal approach helps establish a trigger that switches your mentality away from mundane tasks, such as remembering what's on your to-do list, and into the sacred space of healing. The important thing to remember is that you're emptying out your expectations and attachments so that you can become the clear channel through which Reiki energy flows. Tools like prayer, affirmations, meditation, and reciting the *gokai* can all be excellent triggers for initiating this mind-set. Sincere Reiki practice helps cultivate an authentic heart; remember this when you're beginning your treatments, no matter who the recipient is.

Right Mental Attitude

Although there is no right or wrong way to give Reiki, it's important to remember that you are creating a space for someone's healing. This can mean that whoever is receiving Reiki treatment is entering a vulnerable space as they relax and release. Reiki Ryōhō is compassion in action; the practitioner is practicing kindness and compassion through being fully present and dedicated to the flow of Reiki.

In offering Reiki to yourself and others, it's also important to remember that tension restricts its flow. In this case, tension refers both to physical and psychological tension. In your body, stress and strain can restrict the flow of Reiki to your recipient, just as kinks in a hose inhibit its stream of water. Be sure to be comfortable and at ease during every session. Mentally, do not worry what the outcome will be, as this is a form of strain on the Reiki, too. Just allow yourself to be the empty vessel through which the heart of the universe connects to the heart of your Reiki recipient.

Trying to send Reiki along a specific path can misdirect the energy and prevent it from reaching the cause of a specific condition. In light of this, it's merely enough to place your hands on the recipient and permit Reiki to flow on its own. Recall that *rei* (靈) means "spiritual," "universal," "intelligent," and "effective." Reiki comes from the highest spiritual planes in order to bring healing here and now into our lives. It works universally, and it's guided by its own intelligence.

Being in the right frame of mind may be easy during the initial phase of a Reiki session, but as a practitioner, your mind may wander after prolonged amounts of time. If this is the case, try reciting the *gokai,* or remind yourself to be the empty vessel. You can pray for health, peace, or any other positive outcome, for this will put the mind's efforts to a positive, controlled use.

YOUR REIKI TRIGGER

While specific motions are unnecessary for channeling Reiki, they can be helpful. Any action or set of actions used consistently with the same intention to effect a desired state of mind becomes a mental trigger. Many people begin their Reiki practice by using *gasshō* or another mudra (hand position). In the beginning a practitioner may have to consciously ask to connect to Reiki, but repeated use of your trigger makes the connection automatic and instantaneous.

Gasshō meiso is a specific form of meditation taught by Usui Mikao that, like *gasshō,* brings the two hands together in prayer position at the heart. It is the foundation of virtually every Japanese Reiki Technique, and it is an excellent choice for your personal trigger or protocol. In uniting the hands, you are unifying the polar frequencies of the energy field as well as the mental and spiritual opposites of which we are comprised. Because Reiki in itself is so relaxing and balancing, I sometimes just sit for a moment in *gasshō* whenever I need to clear my mind. (For detailed instructions on how to perform the *gasshō* meditation, please see chapter 8.)

Another form of mental trigger is to use a prayer, affirmation, or mantra when beginning your hands-on practice or a Reiki meditation. The benefit of an affirmation is that it programs the heart-mind to be in a receptive state, and it engages your consciousness while you are in the process of demarcating a space for Reiki. Stating a simple intention or reciting a prayer sets the tone for treatment, and it helps align your actions with the desired outcome of achieving balance through Reiki practice. Here are some helpful affirmations you can try:

- "I am a clear channel for Reiki; Reiki is my guide."
- "I ask my ego and expectations to step aside so Reiki can be my guide."
- "I am a vessel for Reiki. My heart shines its light for healing."
- "May Reiki guide my hands for healing (name the recipient)."
- "I allow Reiki to flow through me for healing (name the recipient)."
- "I align myself with the flow of Reiki; balance, health, and happiness follow effortlessly."
- "I follow the secret way of inviting good fortune. I receive the spiritual medicine of all illness."
- "I accept Reiki. I share Reiki. I am Reiki."
- "I receive and give Reiki freely with compassion and unconditional love."

Similarly, you could merely pray or affirm spontaneously and from the heart. There is no need for a formal process as long as your adherence to Reiki Ryōhō is sincere. Before codifying Usui Reiki Ryōhō as a distinct system, Usui taught his students on a personal basis; everyone received a different set of tools for his or her own growth. It stands to reason that Reiki should be personalized, too, at least to a certain degree. Try creating your own trigger by combining your favorite affirmation with *gasshō,* and watch what happens to your practice.

One of the simplest triggers for initiating the flow of Reiki is merely to ask that it happen. A simple call to the universe is answered unequivocally. Let your request come from a sincere heart, and you will never be disappointed. Reiki will always be there when you ask for it. Don't worry if you aren't able to sense it at first; just content yourself with knowing that it's there.

Ultimately, the only action you need to perform during a Reiki session to start the flow of Reiki is to place your hands where you'd like it to flow. As beautiful as any ritual can be, complex procedures can take away from the simplicity and efficacy of Reiki as a system. Memorizing scripts and choreographed hand movements appeals to the ego, which has difficulty accepting how easy it is to be a conduit for the spiritually guided universal life force. Tame the ego by benching all the tools and techniques you may have learned. Remember the advice of both Hawayo Takata and Yamaguchi Chiyoko: "Hands on, Reiki on! Hands off, Reiki off!"

PRACTICE MAKES PERFECT

As you become more familiar with the motions involved with practicing Reiki, the internal components will flow easily. Doubt and worry will fade away as you grow with Reiki Ryōhō. The easiest way to ensure that your connection to Reiki remains strong is through commitment to regular self-care. You are your own best client, guinea pig, and feedback system. There is nowhere you can go without having access to Reiki, so make time each day to sit with Reiki for self-healing.

Although learning how to get out of your own way mentally can be a challenge, regular practice helps hasten this process. Reiki is mindfulness, and as we place our hands on ourselves, we can really learn to be wholly aware of a single moment. When the mind wanders to your list of unfinished projects or a workplace drama, remind it to come back to Reiki. A simple way to do this is by reflecting on the Reiki precepts; you can even recite them to yourself as you go.

Making a regular habit of treating yourself with Reiki has an added benefit: Not only does your heart-mind surrender more readily, but you also refine your system as a conduit for Reiki. Reiki works by detoxifying. Again, it stirs up what is hidden so that it may be swept away. As we have learned, whenever one practices Reiki for another individual, it first flows through, and therefore heals, the practitioner. The more you give yourself Reiki, the less it theoretically will need to correct or uplift in your own being. This means that you can be more present and more available for your clients, for you will be undeterred by whatever distractions might be going on with your own healing practice. Giving yourself Reiki also means that you are refining and strengthening yourself as a channel for the energy. The more you release, the less there is standing between the source of Reiki and your clients.

I think the best part of this entire process is that you benefit on all levels by committing to being more present for your clients. Giving yourself Reiki ensures your own health and happiness; this makes you a more fully actualized human being who can pay it forward to others. Applying your focus and your skills for the betterment of others (by giving yourself and your clients Reiki) also generates good karma. When you work hard (following the fourth principle: *gyō wo hageme,* or "be diligent in your work"), your meritorious deeds serve everyone.

Reiki is a gift too great to be confined, and it will naturally shine its light on those around you. Using its blessings on yourself teaches you how to connect effortlessly, and it makes you a clearer channel so that you can share Reiki with your loved ones and clients. Practice being mindful and compassionate as you give yourself Reiki, as this will promote a steady stream of healing energy.

Energy Exercises

The best part of teaching the first degree of Reiki is watching new practitioners experience Reiki for the first time. Some practitioners will not have kinesthetic, touchable responses to Reiki, while others may feel various sensations—warmth, tingling, or coolness—as they become a conduit for this spiritual, guided life force. Others might feel a gentle hum in their palms whenever they lay hands on a recipient. It is entirely possible that the practitioner will see, hear, smell, taste, or simply *know* Reiki's flow as he or she practices. However it shows up, it must be greeted lovingly. There is no wrong way to feel Reiki.

Because each of us is predisposed to different skill sets and paradigms, Reiki may manifest itself differently in each person. There is never a need to judge or compare how you connect to Reiki with how anyone else connects. You may need to find your own measure of Reiki flow, but more than likely, with diligent practice, you'll be able to feel what others feel too. This is especially important in the art of sensing *byōsen.* Before learning more about what that is and how you can use it, let's first review some energy-sensing fundamentals.

Try each of the following exercises and see which of them works best for you. You can polish whichever methods produce the weakest results, and you can just as easily maximize your strongest. However you approach them, each one will help you build sensitivity to subtle energies. Take note of what you feel in your hands and body as well as what thoughts arise in your mind. Be sure to refrain from being attached to any outcome or building any specific expectations. It is also fun to compare how sensitive you are before receiving your initiation versus afterward.

❷ Energy Exercise 1: Expanding the Energy

Start by rubbing your hands together vigorously so that they are gently warmed and each of the nerves has been sensitized. Hold your hands in front of you, palm to palm, about one to two inches apart. Mentally ask for Reiki to flow. Wait until you feel it between your palms before progressing. Allow the energy to build until it feels as though your hands are being gently pushed away from one another, as if magnetically repelled.

Allow your hands to drift apart at their own pace. As Reiki flows through and between them, it will fill the space between them. Keep your focus relaxed and just allow the experience to happen. Let the field of energy grow until it is at least one foot in diameter; you could easily let it increase as far as your arms can stretch.

Only spread your palms apart as long as you can still feel the Reiki energy between them. If you are no longer able to sense the field of energy, gently bring your hands together until you can feel it again. Let your palms expand and contract slightly to explore the boundaries of this field of energy. When you are ready to stop, just open your palms until the energy dissipates altogether.

❷ Energy Exercise 2: Directing the Flow of Reiki Energy

As before, begin by rubbing your hands together until they have warmed up. Hold your nondominant hand out with its palm flat. With your other hand point your fingertips toward the palm of your nondominant hand. Visualize energy flowing through your dominant hand and out the fingertips. Gradually bring this hand closer to your outstretched palm until you can feel the beam of energy in the palm of your receptive hand.

Trace a pattern, line, or shape on the palm of your hand from several inches away, as if drawing or painting with Reiki. See how far away your hand can be while the energy remains palpable. After becoming comfortable with how the energy flows, keep moving your hands farther apart. Switch hands and repeat the process. Practice until you can feel the energy on your palm when your hands are more than one foot apart.

This can be an effective training exercise for partners in your class. Pair up and draw on one another's palms with Reiki. See how sensitive you are to your own energy versus that of another person.

❖ Energy Exercise 3: The Energy Ball

Begin this exercise exactly as you began exercise 1. Rub your hands together, extend your palms, and let them expand with the flow of energy. In lieu of expanding them as far as you can, however, stop when they are approximately one foot apart. Once the energy has expanded to fill this space, slowly push your palms toward one another as if compressing the energy between them. Condense it until it reduces in size by one-quarter to one-half. Move your hands around the perimeter of the energy field as if you were polishing a sphere or ball of energy. Palpate the boundaries of the energy ball by moving your hands together and then farther away very slightly.

Once this ball of energy has been formed, you can toss it from hand to hand. Try moving it slowly, then quickly. You can toss it to a partner and see if he or she can feel it as well. Next, holding the orb of Reiki energy in one hand, try using it to trace a line or pattern on the palm of your other hand, as in the second exercise. When finished, you can release the ball upward toward the heavens or send it downward into the ground to heal Mother Earth.

REIKI AS MEDITATION

In the West, Reiki Ryōhō is largely considered to be a hands-on healing method. However, its roots stretch into the arena of spiritual growth and self-realization. If we remember Usui Mikao's personal journey to Reiki, we can see that the goal of Reiki is to help us achieve inner peace, or *anshin ritsumei.* The state of the heart-mind, or *kokoro,* is pivotal in attaining awakening, and meditation is the best way to prepare ourselves for this process.

In the following chapter several specific meditations handed down from Usui's day will be shared. Each has its own goal. Thus you can polish the mirror of your heart-mind with the tools most relevant to your healing journey. However, more generally, anytime you connect to Reiki, you can treat it as a meditation. Whether you choose to engage in *tenohira,* or touch healing, or are merely just reflecting on Reiki itself, Reiki Ryōhō is adaptable to wherever you are and whatever you're doing.

The Reiki Principles gently point us toward an understanding of the nature of mindfulness and its connection to practicing Reiki. As we know, the first injunction in the *gokai* is "today only" or "just for today." This tells us that in order to connect to Reiki, it is necessary to be rooted firmly in the present moment. Steering your awareness back to the eternal now is a valuable tool for any technique you'd like improve, not just Reiki.

Reiki meditation can be formalized or free-form. Practice being mindful of the five admonitions as you recite them each day. You can also use your hands-on healing as a time of honing the mind through meditation. Consciously treating Reiki Ryōhō as a meditative pursuit augments your connection to Reiki during healing overall. Reiki can also support everyday activities as you put your whole heart into them with awareness. Taking a walk, cooking, sipping tea, chanting mantras or affirmations, cleaning, gardening—when undertaking any of these activities we may be inclined to connect with Reiki. Rather than distracting us from the task at hand, Reiki supports our present-moment awareness and links our conscious heart-mind to the power inherent in the now. Note that this is wildly different from the notion of practicing Reiki mindlessly while watching television, eating, or being engaged in other activities. Although we certainly can lay our palms on ourselves or another person during times such as these, the level of mindfulness we access will have a direct effect on the efficacy of our treatment.

The lesson is that connecting to Reiki is an opportunity seeded in each moment of the day. Reiki is not an external force that requires a complicated protocol in order to attract it into our lives; Reiki is omnipresent and aware. It is already within our hearts. Reiki Ryōhō gives us the tools to access it for our continuous evolution and healing.

❖ Reiki Chalice Meditation

It's altogether too easy to think of Reiki as a distinct stream or cord of energy entering the top of your head at the crown chakra during your Reiki practice. Although there is ample literature encouraging you to think this way, a simple visualization can shift this. Rather than only a small diameter of light or energy entering your crown, instead visualize a huge outpouring of Reiki from above. The following exercise can be a simple trigger to incorporate in your personal practice as you connect to Reiki for hands-on treatment.

Sit comfortably and close your eyes. Take several deep breaths and bring your hands together in the *gasshō* position at the heart center. If you use a prayer or affirmation you can recite it now, either silently or aloud. Wait for your hands to give you a signal that Reiki is flowing, such as warmth or a tingling sensation. If no palpable indication arises, trust your intuition.

Now move your hands upward, allowing them to rise and part until your arms are extended in a *V* shape, with your palms ready to cradle the sky. Visualize Reiki coursing into your entire energy field, as if it were filling it entirely. Your arms are raised into a chalice-like shape, signaling to the universe that you are an empty vessel awaiting the infinite blessings of Reiki. Hold this position for a moment as you breathe in the Reiki energy. Sense it passing through the opening of your chalice; let Reiki flow down into your heart through your entire field of light. When you are ready, lower your arms and begin practicing Reiki.

This is a simple exercise that you can repeat as often as you like, either as a stand-alone practice or in conjunction with other techniques. With regular use, the Chalice Meditation will strengthen the flow of Reiki during your meditations and treatments. One of my favorite ways to use it is during the Japanese technique called *reiji hō,* before laying hands on a client or myself. Experiment and find ways to integrate this powerful visualization into your personal practice.

In the next chapter we will more fully explore what is meant by *byōsen,* a form of feedback for the Reiki practitioner. *Byōsen* helps inform the practitioner about what imbalances may exist in a client they are working on. There are different types of *byōsen,* and they all indicate different conditions, as we shall see.

7

UNDERSTANDING *BYŌSEN*

THIS BOOK WAS ORIGINALLY MEANT to be a short guide, a manual if you will, designed in part to teach participants in my Reiki seminars where to find *byōsen* and what it meant. *Byōsen* was the first topic I tackled, and in writing about it, I tried again and again to fit its core concepts into other sections of my written work. However, doing so did not accurately portray the importance of this aspect of Reiki Ryōhō, and because of this, and because *byōsen* can dramatically improve one's practice, I realized that it really deserves its own chapter.

Many Western practitioners are familiar with the term *byōsen* as part of a broader umbrella term—*byōsen reikan hō,* which is the name of a Japanese Reiki Technique. Generally, *byōsen reikan hō* teaches new students that areas of disharmony that exist in the body may be sensed by connecting to Reiki and gently "scanning" above the recipient's body as the practitioner looks for a location to place their hands. (We will learn more about this specific technique of *byōsen reikan hō* in the next chapter.)

This practice is an excellent tool for increasing the efficacy of Reiki treatments because it can lead the practitioner to the underlying cause of a complex condition. However, there is much more to *byōsen* than simply sensing for a spot to touch down. *Byōsen* is a powerful feedback mechanism for the practitioner. It tells you where Reiki is in greatest need. There are different levels of intensity to sensing this energy, and they will point you to the cause of any given illness.

Learning to follow your hands to the strongest *byōsen* requires finesse and practice. In order to develop this sensitivity, Hayashi and Usui both gave their students various exercises and meditations to perform. Takata would urge her students to use Reiki each and every day to reach this level of sensitivity. Practice is genuinely the only way to learn what *byōsen* really is. Once you master it, you will gain a clear understanding of what is happening in the bodies and energy fields of your clients and yourself.

WHAT IS *BYŌSEN?*

Byōsen (病腺) is a concept unique to the original Reiki Ryōhō teachings of Usui Mikao. The word *byōsen* was created by Usui-sensei to describe the sensation of locating areas of disharmony in the client's energy field and body. In Japanese, the word is comprised of the kanji *byō,* 病, signifying "illness" or "sickness," and *sen,* 腺, which translates as "gland" or "lump." Together, the words imply an accumulation, or "lump," of whatever energy or pathology becomes illness. This buildup can be physical, such as toxins within the cells or calcification in the joints, or it can be an accretion of thoughts, emotions, or spiritual energy. Doi Hiroshi, Japanese Reiki practitioner, teacher, and founder of Gendai Reiki, calls *byōsen* "the negative energy generated by the source of disease."[1]

Harnessing *byōsen* during treatment is an exercise in perception. Reiki practitioners can learn to feel *byōsen* through a state of energetic empathy, a form of sympathetic resonance between your energy field and that of the recipient. *Byōsen* is typically experienced as a tangible albeit subtle sensation in the hand or body of the practitioner. This sensation, often termed *hibiki,** is not static; it changes as Reiki is

---

*Some lineages of Reiki Ryōhō substitute the term *hibiki* ("throbbing, tremor") for *byōsen* altogether. This probably began in the 1980s when prominent Reiki figure Doi Hiroshi began to do this, because *byōsen* "sounds like something quasi-medical to postwar Japanese people" (Nishina, *Reiki and Japan,* 140). By avoiding any terminology in this gray area, Reiki practitioners would not be overtly breaking any laws preventing them from practicing.

accepted by the body of the client, leading to a rise and fall, much like the ebb and flow of the tides. These cycles repeat, and they usually show a gradual decrease in intensity over each cycle until the sensation has dissipated.

As we have learned, in the early years of the twentieth century Hayashi Chūjirō branched off from the Usui Reiki Ryōhō Gakkai to develop his own style of practice. Known as the Hayashi Reiki Kenkyukai, this practice was informed by his medical background. One of his greatest contributions to the practice of Reiki was a systematized approach to understanding what *byōsen* is and how it relates to the healing process. Hayashi broke the sensations into five main categories, each representing a specific degree of intensity of the energetic or physical health of the client.

In the *gakkai* it is taught that treatments should continue until *hibiki* dissipates. However, Hayashi discovered that just below *hibiki* was another sensation, called *piri-piri kan.* With this, he discovered that practitioners could improve the efficacy of their treatments by allowing their hands to remain in place until this, too, was released. Hayashi's teachings on *byōsen* have been preserved by the Jikiden Reiki Kenkyukai, thereby making them available to practitioners worldwide.

Through diligent practice (remember the fourth precept: *gyō wo hageme!*) you can learn to discern different levels of energy or *byōsen.* By coupling perception with intuition, you can more effectively treat the core causes of disease and disharmony. When you sense *byōsen,* stick with the current hand position and allow Reiki to dissipate the accumulation of toxins that most likely is present. It nearly always requires longer than the standard five to ten minutes often prescribed in modern branches of the Reiki system.

On the facing page you will find the five major levels of *byōsen* and what they signify to the practitioner. It is important to remember that each practitioner and recipient is unique, and your experience of this energy may be different from another person's. Also, keep in mind that Reiki is not a component of the medical establishment, and thus *byōsen* is not intended to diagnose any person's state of health.

FIVE LEVELS OF *BYŌSEN*

1. Warmth (*onnetsu*, 温熱): This is typically felt as warmer-than-average body temperature. *Onnetsu* indicates that the recipient is receptive to Reiki.

2. Strong warmth (*atsui onnetsu*, 熱い温熱): Stronger heat, such as would make your palms sweat, typically shows that an area may be more depleted or stressed than normal. These are not signs of serious challenges, and they therefore can and should be treated to prevent full-blown problems from developing.

3. Tingling (*piri-piri kan*, ピリピリ感): This is a gentle tingling or pulsing sensation in the hands of the practitioner. Often, *piri-piri kan* is a sign that illness may be developing. Generally, this level of *byōsen* will gradually decrease within two or three cycles.

4. Throbbing (*hibiki*, 響き): Similar to level three, the fourth stage of *byōsen* has a pulsing or throbbing sensation; in this instance it is much stronger and more persistent. Sometimes *hibiki* will extend beyond the hand and creep along the practitioner's arm. Level four *byōsen* clearly indicates an area in need of Reiki; it is often accompanied by pain, fatigue, or illness in the client. Allow your hands to stay in place at least until *hibiki* (level four) has reduced to *atsui onnetsu* (level two, strong heat). My teacher Frank Arjava Petter indicated that *hibiki* is almost always a sign of inflammation or infection. It may require several treatments to resolve. Occasionally, throbbing will give way to a coldness or heaviness, which can be considered halfway between levels four and five.

5. Pain (*itami*, 痛み): Level five *byōsen* is described as pain, discomfort, or heaviness. In many healing systems we are taught that the healer should never experience pain or discomfort; otherwise they are taking on the condition of the client. With Reiki, the initiation awakens our energetic sensitivity, which enables us to better perceive the client's state of being. Therefore, when we feel *itami,* or pain, in our hands and bodies, it is *not* that we are

taking on the illness of our clients. *Itami* only points the way to the most serious accumulation of toxic or imbalanced energy in the recipient's makeup. Level five *byōsen* can vary in intensity, sometimes traveling along the Reiki practitioner's arm and shoulder and down the side of the body.

HOW *BYŌSEN* DEVELOPS

The word *byōsen* refers to two related concepts. It describes the cause of illness or discomfort, which is the accumulation of physical or energetic patterns that are toxic. *Byōsen* also describes the body's reaction to receiving Reiki treatment, which is responsible for the subtle sensations of rising and falling felt in the practitioner's hands and body.

In Japan there is a phrase that describes the body's natural cleansing process: *shizen jōka sayō* (自然浄化作用).[2] This translates roughly to "natural purification action" or "natural cleansing process," and it is a term used in medical and natural healing modalities alike. In the philosophy of *shizen jōka sayō,* the body is continuously processing toxins from the diet, environment, and internal processes. Our feelings affect the chemistry of our body as a result of the hormonal secretions that are stimulated by our various emotional states. Overall, a healthy system can effectively dispose of toxic energy or substances by placing—in strategic locations in the body—anything that it cannot eliminate on its own. This prevents systemic toxicity.[3]

Whenever the body's function has been disrupted, such as by stress, fatigue, diet, environment, or other factors, these deposits of unhealthy or disharmonious buildup cannot be properly eliminated. As more of this toxicity is accreted, *byōsen* increases in intensity. When we add Reiki energy to the body of a client, we are providing the fuel that is necessary to tackle the removal of those unhealthy deposits. The movement of this energy stirs the body's natural elimination process—*shizen jōka sayō*—which can be perceived by the Reiki practitioner as the ebb and flow of *byōsen.*

The average body accumulates *byōsen* according to a principle called *heikin jōka* (平均浄化), which means "balanced cleansing."[4] Like *shizen jōka sayō, heikin jōka* is not a term unique to Reiki. Balanced cleansing in this context means that *byōsen* accrues in roughly equal measure on opposite parts of the body. Since it is accumulated more or less symmetrically, an injured or painful knee or shoulder, for example, will also result in the storage of toxins in and around the unaffected half of the matching pair. Reiki should be offered to both sides of the body, if possible, especially for long-standing conditions.

WHERE *BYŌSEN* LURKS

During a Reiki treatment you may find *byōsen* virtually anywhere. These sensations can result from physical illness or injury as well as the behavior, beliefs, and feelings held by your client. Reiki heals them all, no matter their level of existence. *Byōsen* is your most valuable feedback tool, especially when you can anticipate where to find it.

The most obvious places to find *byōsen* include the site of an injury, surgery, trauma, or illness. However, sometimes the body compensates for the outer symptoms, which can lead to sensations of *byōsen* in seemingly unrelated places. For example, an injured ankle will surely produce level four or level five *byōsen;* however, the hip and knee on the opposite leg are likely to have *byōsen* that is nearly as intense because they are compensating for the painful or tender ankle. Again, whenever you encounter injuries, be sure to seek *byōsen* on the opposite side of the body.

Usually the body is able to process all of its toxins on its own. It may occasionally store these in benign areas until they can be later mitigated or released. Some predictable places in which this stored *byōsen* can be felt include:

- shoulders and shoulder blades
- hips and glutes
- throat
- kidneys and adrenal glands
- intestines

- the upper, middle, and lower *tanden:* brow, heart, and *hara*
- lower back
- knees
- lymph nodes
- the head: sinuses, temples, back of the head[5]

Additional *byōsen* can often be felt in locations where injury has occurred, among the internal organs, and often in the feet, which, in modalities such as reflexology, serve as a map of the entire body. A friend and colleague of mine who is both a Reiki practitioner and a reflexologist is often able to pinpoint issues in the body just by treating the feet. She senses the *byōsen* in specific points on the feet, which indicate impacted areas of the body.

It is not uncommon to feel *byōsen* in the aura or chakras, especially when performing *byōsen reikan hō* (described in the next chapter). Mental or emotional *byōsen* can frequently be felt at the head and heart, but it is possible for them to manifest elsewhere, too. Sometimes the underlying cause of an illness or condition is largely nonphysical. In cases such as these, we may feel mild *byōsen* where the symptoms manifest, whereas the more intense *byōsen* (such as *hibiki* or *itami)* manifest at the site of the condition's cause.

If there are multiple locations in which *byōsen* is found, it's likely that several treatments are needed to ameliorate all of them. You as a practitioner can try to feel out or intuit the most effective places to start, or you may refer to the *reiji hō* method found in the following chapter. This will permit you to treat *byōsen* strategically, beginning with the areas that are the most critical or time-sensitive. If you target the most serious areas first, the body can assist in alleviating areas of lesser degrees of intensity on its own.

HELPFUL TIPS

Remember that *byōsen* depends on your ability to be the empty vessel; there is no need to do any "work" when practicing Reiki Ryōhō. Allow

Reiki to be your guide and it will help you develop the sensitivity to these states through daily practice. The more you use Reiki, the more sensitive your hands become! Some of the Japanese Reiki Techniques, including *hatsurei hō,* are able to enhance your perception of *byōsen,* too.

The body itself has many different rhythmic forces that can be conflated with *byōsen.* The pulse of the circulatory system can be deceptive. This is because both the practitioner's and client's pulses may be mistaken for *hibiki.* The activity of the digestive system and the circulatory system and the movement of lymph and secretions from the glands may each contribute sensations of their own during a session. Reiki practitioners can attain discernment between *byōsen* and these mechanical movements through practice and patience. Remember that the energy sensed as *byōsen* is a subtle rather than physical aspect of Reiki treatment.

Other sensations often experienced as part of *byōsen* may include attraction, repulsion, cold, hollowness, heaviness, flux or flow, and/or even itchiness. See what each means by watching the rise and fall of the energy and mentally comparing these sensations to the five basic levels of *byōsen.* Beginning students often feel *byōsen* in their bodies, rather than their hands, and it is typically easier to detect *byōsen* in others than in ourselves.

To test whether the sensation is yours or your client's, gently lift the palm of your hand off the body of your client, with fingertips maintaining light contact. If the sensation disappears, it is *byōsen*; if it does not, it might be necessary to adjust your position so that these sensations are ameliorated and you remain comfortable for the duration of the Reiki treatment.

In the successive degrees of Reiki training, practitioners are introduced to the sacred symbols used in Reiki Ryōhō. One of these augments the flow of energy and directs its focus to the target area, which makes it ideal for treating the *byōsen* felt in your client's body or energy field. For this reason, many practitioners advance to *okuden* to enhance their practice.*

---

*In Jikiden Reiki, *shirushi* for targeting *byōsen* is taught in the final part of *shoden* training. Most styles of Reiki Ryōhō reserve all the symbols (*shirushi* and *jumon*) for the *okuden* seminar.

TREATING *BYŌSEN* WITH REIKI

Although placing a hand anywhere will allow Reiki to flow into the recipient, learning how to target the most effective zone can dramatically improve results and reduce treatment duration. Ideally, treatments must continue until the *byōsen* has been reduced or eliminated altogether. Following your intuition is one of the best ways to do this, and regular practice will help you hone this skill set.

When introducing practitioners to *byōsen* for the first time, I liken it to approaching a dark canyon. Placing our hands on the client is like tossing a pebble into that deep crevice. We may have to wait some time for the stone to reach the bottom, but when it does we can learn valuable information about the depth and width of the canyon based on the echo it produces. Likewise, when we place our hands over a specific area of the body, the *byōsen* may not be immediately perceptible. You must wait for the sensations to arise or you run the risk of walking away without hearing the echo at all. In this way we can understand the severity of our client's conditions. If we can exercise patience, we are almost always guaranteed to find at least a lower-level sensation arising from *byōsen*. If we are impatient, then we will surely miss even the most intense levels altogether.

Again, *byōsen* works by stirring up toxic accumulations. These stored toxins can be physical in nature, or they may be toxic thoughts, emotions, behaviors, and energies. Hayashi-sensei used to describe how *byōsen* works by using the analogy of a muddy stream.[6] The stored energies are akin to the silty, muddy bottom of the stream. Practicing Reiki and enacting *byōsen* is like stirring a stream that appears crystal clear; reaching into the bottom of the stream and moving the mud makes the waters turbid and dark. After a short while, the natural flow of the stream sweeps the silty deposits downstream in order to clear them away. As we have established, the body works in this same fashion to remove and detoxify the hidden energy or materials that have been brought to light through the action of Reiki. As we leave our hands in place, Reiki penetrates deeper and deeper, stirring more mud in the metaphorical stream each time. Eventually, the bottom of the stream is clean and clear, and the flow of the water is completely unimpeded by the previous accumulation. This is how Reiki supports the body's natural equilibrium.

Hawayo Takata did not use the term *byōsen,* although it is evident that she urged her students to follow their hands.* Takata-sensei is quoted as saying, "Reiki will guide you. Let the Reiki hands find it. They will know what to do."[7] This is the essence of *byōsen* even if it's not addressed by its original name.

Takata taught her students to give a complete treatment, which she called the Foundation Treatment. This basic pattern of hand positions ensured that the practitioner's touch would reach each major organ of the body, as well as nourishing and healing the subtle anatomy. The Foundation Treatment itself is a starting point; before you are sensitive enough to feel *byōsen,* using this method means that you will automatically target the most important spots. As you become more sensitized, you will likely stay longer and longer in spots where you feel *byōsen* lurking.

Harry Kuboi was one of Takata's twenty-two *shihan*. He describes, in his writings on Reiki, the process of finding *byōsen:* "Reiki is a very simple method of helping people with physical problems. Wherever a person puts his hands, his hands can begin to pick up sensations—tingling, burning, numbing—indicating that there is congestion in that area."[8] The sensations that he is describing are clearly *byōsen,* which tells us that Takata understood and taught the nuances of these energetic sensations. Mr. Kuboi also tells us, "Treating the whole body for a specific problem is not productive. First of all find a person's specific problem. One needs to find the CAUSE in order to remove the EFFECT."[9]

---

*It's likely that Takata-sensei avoided stressing the concept of *byōsen* for the same reason that the founder of Gendai Reiki, Doi Hiroshi, substited *hibiki* for the term: to avoid breaking laws regarding unlicensed medical practice. Given that Takata initially practiced and taught Reiki Ryōhō in a time when anti-Japanese sentiment was high, she also streamlined and Westernized much of the system of Reiki, which must have influenced how she approached *byōsen*.

The "CAUSE" to which Kuboi-sensei refers is the area in which the strongest *byōsen* can be felt. These feelings, especially level four (throbbing or *hibiki*) and level five (pain or *itami*) can travel beyond the hand, extending up the arm and down the side of the body of the practitioner. Harry indicated that these sensations are perfectly normal, much like his teacher Mrs. Takata surely did, and felt that they did not reflect a transference of energy between practitioner and client.[10]

Although any Reiki is better than no Reiki at all, learning to treat the cause of disharmony through sensitivity to *byōsen* will change your practice dramatically. Spending an hour or more on a single location is not unheard of as you allow Reiki to completely penetrate the core of the congested, stagnant energy in order to release it. Practice "listening" to *byōsen* with your hands as you practice on yourself and your clients.

RECOGNIZING PATTERNS IN *BYŌSEN*

As we become acquainted with sensing *byōsen* in our clients, there will be some distinct patterns to the rise and fall of these sensations that may become familiar. Even though there are exceptions to every rule, one typically finds that acute conditions have similar patterns, just as chronic and terminal cases will exhibit similar *byōsen*. Some healers have even noted that the particular pattern or degree of intensity exhibited by clients can be a clear indication of exactly what type of illness they have; it is as though the diseases have a signature *byōsen* that identifies them.*

The most commonly encountered pattern of *byōsen* is illustrated at the top of the facing page. This pattern is typical of long-standing conditions that have not yet manifested as symptoms of outright illness or imbalance. The cycles are slow, gentle, and sometimes stubborn. Because this disharmony has usually formed over time, at least three to five sessions to reduce or eliminate the *byōsen* altogether may be

---

*For more graphs depicting the cycles of *byōsen* please see *This Is Reiki* by Frank Arjava Petter (page 197) and *Light on the Origins of Reiki* by Yamaguchi Tadao (page 76).

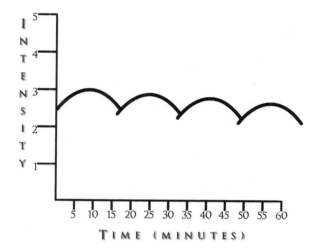

Byōsen of an unmanifest condition; note its cyclical highs and lows

required. Although the energy may soon sink to a level two or three *byōsen* (meaning "heat" or "tingling"), it is likely to rise again after the first treatment. The key is to treat repeatedly over the course of several days or weeks until the *byōsen* finally dissipates.

The graph below represents patterns of acute illness or injury. The cycles respond to Reiki treatment within two or three short cycles that

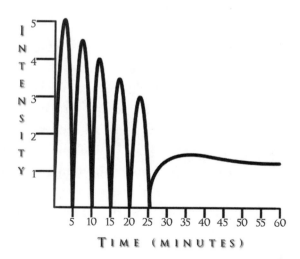

Byōsen of an acute condition, featuring cyclical extremes

crest very quickly. Over the course of a single treatment they are likely to taper off. As we have indicated previously but bears repeating here, if this category of *byōsen* isn't treated right away, it can lead to full-blown illness or a chronic imbalance. Cold and flu detected early often have this pattern of *byōsen,* as do minor injuries. Treat continuously until the waves of *byōsen* diminish below level three; this can usually be attained within two or three treatments for colds, or a single session for a simple injury.

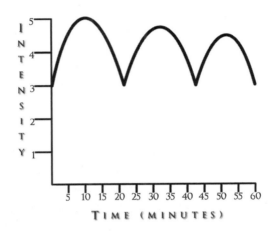

Byōsen of a chronic condition, which will require
several sessions of treatment to resolve

Byōsen such as the pattern depicted above accompanies chronic illness and pain, which may be the result of an injury or disease that has not fully healed. The *byōsen* in these scenarios can be tenacious; they may seem to resist treatment for several sessions, often returning exactly to the starting point in a gradual process after each session. Regular treatment over the course of weeks may be necessary to relieve this type of *byōsen* of its intensity and frequency. Try treating your client once each day for four or five days in a row, then reduce treatment to once or twice a week until conditions improve. This kind of *byōsen* also responds well to the concentrated energy of group treatments as well as the distance treatment learned in *okuden,* or the second degree.

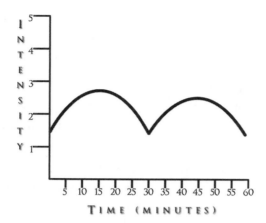

Byōsen in a healthy person, featuring regular cycles that
are not extreme in nature

The figure above illustrates the *byōsen* of a fairly healthy person. Note that it is relatively slow-moving, but it does not peak very high. This is typically the type of energy felt when a healthy body merely needs a little replenishing through Reiki.

Byōsen that remains at level five or level four over a sustained period of time indicates a serious condition or a terminal illness. Late-stage cancer patients often create a constant *itami* (pain) sensation in the hands and bodies of practitioners. In these cases, although Reiki can and often

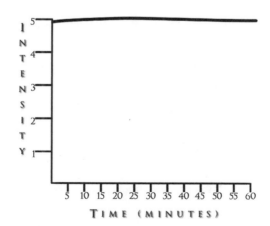

Byōsen of a critical or terminal illness remains
at an intense level over a sustained period

will work miracles, it will just as often be a gentle part of the transition process for the ill individual. Constant level five *byōsen* can sometimes be uncomfortable for practitioners, so if you are treating someone with this type of *byōsen,* be sure to take breaks or switch hands to complete the Reiki treatment so you don't stretch yourself too far. The symbols and other tools in the second degree can help in this process.

Byōsen changes over time, especially after successive Reiki treatments. Pay attention to how the patterns have changed and what you have done to treat them each time. Keeping notes about treatments can give you valuable insights into what to do with future clients in similar situations. Remember to practice on yourself, and pay attention to how the *byōsen* in your own body changes over time as well.

ANIMALS AND *BYŌSEN*

Little information on the *byōsen* felt in animals has been published to date. Hayashi's teachings did not include treatments for animals, and it is likely that the Usui Reiki Ryōhō Gakkai did not record the *byōsen* of animals either. As a result, we are left to make observations and draw conclusions on our own about the nature of *byōsen* in the animal kingdom.

Generally speaking, it has been my experience that smaller animals have much more rapid cycles of *byōsen* than larger animals do. It stands to reason that, since the rest of their biological processes have faster cycles, their *byōsen* would follow suit. I have treated rodents extensively, and it is often difficult to perceive any *byōsen* at all unless chronic or terminal conditions are present. Larger animals, on the other hand, exhibit much slower patterns of *byōsen.*

It is usually much easier to treat most animals with hands-off or distance treatments. Without the *okuden* training and the subsequent *jumon* used in distance healing, however, it may initially be challenging to perceive *byōsen* during hands-off treatments. Diligent practice will allow you to discern these cycles over time. When giving treatments from a short distance away from an animal, it is as likely that you will feel the sensations in your body as in your hands. In my experience, with remote treatments such as *enkaku chiryō,* described on page 271, practitioners will perceive *byōsen* much more readily in their hands.

Animal Reiki experts Elizabeth Fulton and Kathleen Prasad suggest that when treating animals, the practitioner remains in position until any physical sensations subside, just as one would do when treating people. They go on to remind practitioners to "weigh the physical information you receive [i.e., *byōsen*] in light of other factors, such as the animal's appearance and behavior, your own intuitive sense of the situation, and any information you have from the animal's person, if the animal is not your own companion."[11] Since animals are unable to communicate and provide feedback in the way that adult humans can, pay close attention to the *byōsen* and frame it within the context of all the other information you have.

Monitoring the *byōsen* of animals you are treating will deepen the efficacy of treatments, as is true for human beings also. Keep your mind in a relaxed state of awareness, and surrender to the flow of Reiki during the treatment. Reiki will do the rest.

❖ Byōsen Graphing

Create a blank graph or copy the one on the following page and use it to monitor *byōsen* during your own treatments. Locate an area on your body (or in your energy field) where you usually find *byōsen,* and treat it with Reiki. Keep a watch or clock nearby so you can make some mental notes about how long each *byōsen* cycle lasts. When it has diminished or been eliminated altogether, draw out the curves of each cycle; be sure to include the level of intensity as well as the approximate duration of each cycle. Some important ideas to keep in mind while practicing include:

- At what level does the *byōsen* begin?
- At what level does the *byōsen* reach its peak?
- Are the two sides of each curve symmetrical, or does it rise faster or more slowly than it falls?

- Do the cycles last for the same amount of time, or do they shorten during the course of treatment?
- Do you know the underlying cause of the *byōsen,* such as an old injury or habitual illness?

With regular practice, you can start to anticipate how *byōsen* will respond to Reiki. This enables you to adapt your hand positions and other tools that you employ in order to better reach into the causal level of disease instead of merely treating the symptoms. More than one root cause can influence *byōsen,* including the attitude, beliefs, and lifestyle of the recipient. Over time, you can encourage your clients to adjust these variables in order to facilitate healing at the core level.

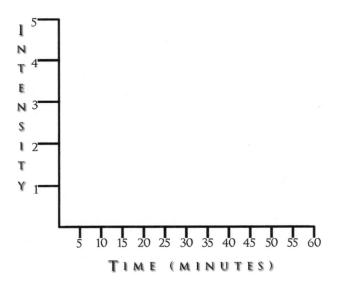

A blank graph for charting *byōsen*

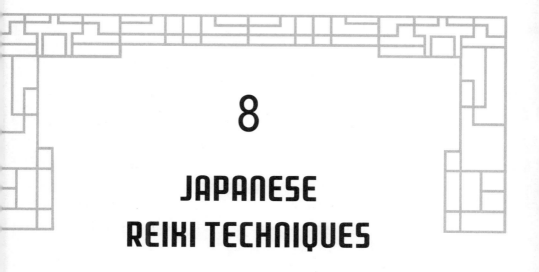

8

JAPANESE
REIKI TECHNIQUES

GIVEN THAT REIKI ORIGINATED IN JAPAN, some of its practices and methodologies are uniquely Japanese in character. These include various means of connecting to Reiki, enhancing the flow of Reiki for treatment, and various protocols to employ for treatment itself. In addition, most of the meditative procedures have an overtly spiritual quality, pointing us toward the core of the Reiki system as being spiritually—not physically—oriented.

The Japanese Reiki Techniques, or *Nihon no Reiki gihō* (日本の技法), have gained popularity among many different lineages of Reiki. They impart a feeling of authenticity and a connection to Usui himself. These methods are a means of cultivating our inner connection to Reiki, and they will help improve our skills in administering Reiki overall. Usui taught these *gihō* to enable his students to advance; we can use them today with similar results.

HISTORICAL BACKGROUND

Usui-sensei introduced most of the techniques below, and his successors at the Usui Reiki Ryōhō Gakkai preserved them in each succeeding generation. Like all living traditions, the practice of Reiki Ryōhō has evolved; some of the Japanese Reiki Techniques have changed over time and new methods have also been adopted. Hayashi and his students practiced many of the following methods, although often in slightly modified forms. Even Hawayo Takata used many of the techniques in this chapter; she typically presented them without their original names, however.

The following tools and practices have a pronounced Japanese character. Some of them, such as *kenyoku hō,* conjure the rituals of purification used at Buddhist temples and Shinto shrines in Japan. The memorial stone at Usui's grave tells us that he studied a variety of spiritual practices, including native Japanese traditions and some from outside Japan, like Christianity. There are also close parallels between some of the *gihō* practices used in qigong (called *kiko* in Japanese). Because of his personal background, Usui Mikao distilled the best methods he encountered into the formation of Reiki Ryōhō.

After Usui, Hayashi's school, the Hayashi Reiki Kenkyukai, and various teachers connected to the Usui Reiki Ryōhō Gakkai and those teaching independently would continue to propagate the Japanese Reiki Techniques. This work is continued in several other branches of Reiki in Japan, including Gendai Reiki Hō and Jikiden Reiki, as well as many Western organizations, including the International Center for Reiki Training in Michigan and many independent Reiki teachers. Over the years these methods have occasionally been updated, with a newer technique appearing here and there while the original *gihō* remained intact.

One final note before introducing these techniques themselves: in Japan, practitioners usually sit in a position known as *seiza,* or 正座, which means "correct sitting." One kneels on the floor and sits on one's heels; the big toes are usually lightly crossed. If this position is uncomfortable for any reason, the techniques may be tried with the practitioner seated in a chair or standing.

THE THREE PILLARS

The *gakkai* preaches a threefold approach to Reiki practice, which they call the Three Pillars of Reiki.[1] These pillars are *gasshō, reiji hō,* and *chiryō.* Together, these three aspects of Reiki represent the three avenues by which we may improve ourselves through the practice. *Gasshō* is the joining of the hands in a prayerful state. Its formal meditation technique is outlined below; it's called *gasshō meiso. Reiji hō* allows the consciousness of Reiki to guide the hands; it helps prepare the intuition. Finally, *chiryō* simply means "treatment" or "therapy." This is the hands-on application of Reiki that is learned in the first degree.

If we examine the Three Pillars a little more closely, we see that they work together on the threefold aspects of our being: heart-mind, spirit, and body. Usui maintained that his therapy was primarily oriented toward healing and training the nonphysical parts of one's being; therefore *gasshō* and *reiji hō* precede *chiryō.*

Gasshō brings awareness to the heart center. When the hands are brought together before the heart, the goal is to let go and become as empty as possible. This meditation calms and clears the conscious mind, so that the sincere heart can shine through. It is this inner heart-mind that represents our real awareness of the self. *Gasshō* makes it possible to polish our awareness of this part of ourself. It balances polarities as represented by the two hands coming together, and it trains the mind to be a vessel for spirit.

Reiji hō, or "the method of indicating by spirit," moves the hands to the brow. We pray for guidance to come to us in such a way that it guides the hands exactly to where Reiki is most needed by the recipient. Using this method can only be genuinely helpful once the conscious mind is made quiet and aligned with spirit. *Reiji hō* helps us actualize our spiritual nature. It deepens the intuition and serves as a bridge between the physical or outer aspect that receives Reiki and the spiritual or inner aspect from which Reiki originates.

Finally, *chiryō,* or treatment, rounds out the Three Pillars. This is simply putting Reiki into practice. We can treat ourselves, our loved ones, our pets, our food, our goals, or nearly anything else if we use enough imagination. *Chiryō* nourishes the physical body and it signals to the spirit that Reiki is needed when we administer our gentle, loving touch. *Chiryō* is a form of "doing without doing" because, again,

Reiki practitioners do not need to focus or direct Reiki energy.

Together the Three Pillars help nourish and heal all three aspects of the self. They are the three inroads to health and balance through which Reiki moves. Making them a daily practice helps train your "Reiki muscles" so that you can polish your heart-mind until it reflects your luminous spirit and nothing short of that.

REINCORPORATING THE JAPANESE TECHNIQUES

Although these practices have been reintroduced to the Westernized branches of Reiki, Takata-sensei clearly taught many of these methods simply, without referring to them by their original names. This is because her audience consisted primarily of speakers of English.[2] Her diary indicates that she learned these techniques, including *reiji hō,* when she studied under Hayashi-sensei. She called *reiji hō* "the utmost in the energy science."[3]

In the 1990s, Frank Arjava Petter began the process of training Western practitioners in the *Nihon no Reiki gihō,* the Japanese Reiki Techniques. Through the tireless work of many influential writers and Reiki *shihan,* we have seen these methods spread far and wide. Many popular Reiki manuals, such as those written by prominent Reiki practitioner and author William Lee Rand (*Reiki: The Healing Touch*), have incorporated many of the Japanese techniques so that they can be reintegrated into modern healing methods. Several Japanese instructors, like Doi Hiroshi, continue to spread the teachings, thus granting an authentic Japanese connection among the practices of Reiki lovers worldwide.

While many teachers do offer insight and instruction into the Japanese Reiki Techniques, many do not. Given that the exercises have been translated from one culture to many others, they have also been adapted, distorted, and otherwise altered from generation to generation. I'll attempt to keep them as simple and authentic as possible below. (Readers interested in deepening their understanding of the Japanese

Reiki Techniques can find additional materials containing information about them in the bibliography.) Although the majority of the following tools date back to Usui and Hayashi, a couple of them are newer additions to the Reiki toolbox. Experiment and see which ones work best for you.

❖ Gasshō Meiso 合掌瞑想

The first of the Three Pillars of Reiki Ryōhō as outlined by the Usui Reiki Ryōhō Gakkai is *gasshō*. *Gasshō* is written with the kanji for "unite" (合) and "palm" (掌); it literally signifies, as we have learned, bringing the palms of the hands together as a symbol of reverence or piety. *Meiso* simply means "meditation." This Japanese Reiki Technique is the foundation of most of the following exercises. Spending a few moments in *gasshō* stills the mind, alleviates stress, and centers one's whole being.

Each of the fingers on each hand can be representative of the different aspects of one's being. For example, they can be associated with the five elements of Eastern philosophy and medicine (wood, water, fire, earth, and metal); they can also represent the five elements of traditional or alchemical lore (fire, water, air, earth, and spirit/ether/akasha). The hands, in Buddhism and other Asian worldviews, also relate to our archetypal opposites. The right hand is active, giving, solar, open, and *yang*. Left, on the other hand, is thus symbolic of being passive, receptive, lunar, closed (or hidden), and *yin*. To bring together these opposing forces in the stillness of meditation offers us total balance; this act harmonizes our elemental nature and offers reconciliation between opposing energies.

When the hands are brought together, they are usually held at the heart or just above it. The height at which one's hands are placed traditionally reflects the amount of reverence or respect being shown. Since *gasshō* isn't being used as a gesture or greeting, heart level is sufficient for Reiki purposes. The palms are usually held together, although some teachers recommend a small gap between them. The fingertips are united, with the most emphasis placed on the middle finger.

As you practice *gasshō meiso,* the idea is merely to still the mind and empty yourself of attachment and expectation. Thoughts will naturally come up; this is completely normal. Even practiced meditators often experience this. The trick is to just observe them as they pass, rather than follow them wherever they may be trying to lead. An easy trick is just to imagine stepping back and looking at your thoughts from farther away. If you try to resist or erase your thinking, you will encounter resistance. Just relax and allow.

The effects of *gasshō meiso* include sharper focus and greater ease when channeling Reiki. Each of the fingers is related to a different meridian, or energy channel, in the body. Bringing them together helps them work in perfect balance. This serves as a way to prime the pumps, so that when you engage in other meditative or healing methods you will be a clearer vessel for Reiki to pass through.

When you are practicing *gasshō,* bring your awareness to your middle finger; this is the finger associated with the element of fire. It is the power finger. Traditional Reiki, also referred to as *dento Reiki* in Japan, recognizes it as the most potent of the fingers when Reiki is applied for hands-on healing. Gently directing your attention to the place where the tips of your middle fingers meet gives your mind a means of avoiding attachment to arising thoughts. It also helps generate an affinity for the archetype of fire, which is cleansing and warming. This meditative experience can ignite the spark of healing and spiritual growth that underlies all of the practices in Reiki Ryōhō.

Initially, try practicing *gasshō* in silence for five minutes or so. Over time you can stretch this to as long as thirty minutes or an hour. Diligent meditation helps train the mind and spirit, your *kokoro.* This is the real goal of Usui Reiki Ryōhō, and *gasshō* is the first tool we learn in order to begin the process of awakening to our true selves. Usui even asks us to practice *gasshō meiso* twice each day while reciting the precepts: *asa yū gasshō shite kokoro ni nenji kuchi ni tona e yo* ("morning and evening practice *gasshō* and hold [the principles] in your heart and chant them with your mouth"[4]).

The more you practice *gasshō,* the easier it will be. Since it is the first part of most of the techniques and is even used during *reiju,* most practitioners feel Reiki flow whenever they place their palms together at the heart. This makes *gasshō* a perfect trigger for connecting to the flow of Reiki, as discussed in chapter 6. Committing to a regular practice of *gasshō* helps polish the mirror of the heart, and it embodies the fourth precept, *gyō wo hageme,* which invites us to work with diligence toward uncovering our authentic selves.

1. Sit comfortably and set your intention to meditate. Traditionally, this meditation is practiced in *seiza,* the Japanese manner of sitting, which is a kneeling position with the feet tucked beneath the body. Feel free to sit in a chair or cross-legged on the ground.
2. Bring your hands together in front of the heart. Allow for a minute amount of space between the palms, with the fingers together in "prayer position."
3. Bring your awareness to the point where the middle fingertips meet. When thoughts arise, simply observe them detachedly; neither pursue nor dismiss them.
4. Continue meditating in this fashion until you are unable to continue or until you've drawn the exercise to a close.

❂ Kenyoku Hō 乾浴法

The kanji in *kenyoku hō* translate to "dry bathing method." This is a simple energetic activity designed to cleanse the practitioner before and after hands-on healing. It consists of sweeping Reiki-charged palms across the body and down the arms. Imagine that it is similar to dusting off any disharmonious energy, much like you are sweeping the energy field and meridians clear. The practice is similar in idea to the concept of *temizu,* a handwashing ceremony practiced before one enters shrines and temples in Japan.

The rhythm of this exercise is decidedly Japanese; practicing the sweeps with an odd-numbered pattern adheres to the Japanese aesthetic and is in keeping with the *temizu* ceremony. Both *kenyoku hō* and *temizu* belong to a family of practices, originating from Shinto, called *harae.* *Harae* are rituals of purification that are meant to eliminate the uncleanness that we acquire from living in this world. *Kenyoku* serves to help us leave behind our bad habits, limiting thinking, disharmony, and impure vibrations.

The unequal patterns used in this technique and the sweeping motion employed are similar to some exercises taught in qigong. It is likely that Reiki Ryōhō founder Usui Mikao adapted what he learned into the practice of Reiki in order to give practitioners a means of energetically cleansing themselves in preparation for administering Reiki to others.

Kenyoku hō can be used before placing your hands on a client or yourself. It is also a simple and effective method of releasing any echo of the energy left by your clients *after* a Reiki treatment. The simplicity of this exercise makes it easy to learn and use in public venues, such as at Reiki circles and Reiki shares, wherein practitioners often move directly from one recipient to the next. *Kenyoku* can even be used after an upsetting or unpleasant experience in order to sweep away the energies left by such events.

Intention and visualization enhance the effects of this meditation. By beginning in *gasshō,* you trigger the automatic response necessary to engage the flow of Reiki energy. As you continue through the rest of the exercise, visualizing energy or light flowing through the palms of the hands as they are swept across the body helps support the end goal of cleansing. When I first learned this technique, my *shihan* encouraged us to sweep the discordant vibrations into a candle flame or the glow of a salt lamp. Although I believe that Reiki serves to transmute any disharmonious energy, this additional step can promote an even more effective cleansing.

1. Begin in *gasshō*. Wait until you feel Reiki flowing before proceeding.
2. Place your right hand on your left shoulder. Sweep diagonally down and across your body to your right hip.
3. Reverse hands. With your left hand on your right shoulder, sweep down to your left hip.
4. Repeat step 2.
5. Place your right hand on your left shoulder. Sweep down your left arm and hand.
6. Move your left hand to your right shoulder and sweep down the right arm and hand.
7. Repeat step 5.
8. End with a brief *gasshō*.

❂ Reiki Shower 靈氣シャワー

The Reiki Shower is a technique popularized in the system of Gendai Reiki Hō taught by Doi Hiroshi.[5] It can serve as an adjunct to or replacement of *kenyoku hō*. The Reiki Shower exercise served as the original inspiration for the

Reiki Chalice Meditation found in chapter 6. Doi writes that the "Reiki Shower cleanses the physical body and activates the energy body by absorbing Reiki energy throughout the body like a shower."[6] Similar practices may also be part of the *gakkai*'s teachings.

My initial introduction to this technique occurred when my very first Reiki teacher returned from having studied with Doi-sensei himself. She added this to her class syllabus, and it became one of my favorite tools in my Reiki toolbox. It also serves to remind us that we don't simply receive Reiki from the top of the head; rather, Reiki inundates the entire energy field as it streams into and through the practitioner. As this happens, the entire body will feel saturated with Reiki, leaving us refreshed and ready to practice.

1. While standing or sitting, quiet the mind and practice *gasshō*.
2. Raise your arms above the head so that they form a *V* shape. Allow Reiki to flow through your energy field, and take note of how it emanates from your palms.
3. As the Reiki is flowing, slide the palms of your hands downward through your energy field, directing them toward the front (or sides) of your body. Move them deliberately and smoothly from head to toe. Allow Reiki to flow through them and clear away any vibrations in need of release.
4. End with *gasshō*.

❖ *Reiji Hō* 靈示法

As the second of the Three Pillars, *reiji hō* is a powerful tool for accessing your intuition in order to find the most effective place to treat a client. Takata-sensei once described this as the pinnacle of the techniques she learned from her teacher. *Reiji* is comprised of two kanji; the first is the same *rei* in *Reiki,* whereas *ji* (示) translates as "to show" in modern Japanese. Together, the expression *reiji hō* means "method of being shown by spirit." In our practice we could really translate this as "being shown by Reiki," for it is a tool for connecting to the consciousness of Reiki in order to treat the origin of disease.

In Japanese, the expression 病元 or *byōgen* means "the origin of disease." Although Reiki is an intelligent force that can find its way to the underlying concerns, it sometimes works very slowly as it makes its way through other areas of disharmony in need of resolution. *Reiji hō* is a means of accessing the guiding force of Reiki in order to point the practitioner, in a more directed way, toward the *byōgen,* or origin of the scenario. This technique is especially helpful when the cause is unknown, when there are confusing or conflicting conditions, or when someone is in otherwise good health and wants to be treated to maintain that state.

After beginning in *gasshō,* you will move your hands upward to the brow and set the intention that Reiki will guide the hands. This can be a short prayer or affirmation, or it can just be a silent feeling. You must sincerely want to work for the wellness and happiness of your client in order to achieve results. After getting into the right state of mind, you must simply wait for an answer to the call.

Most of the time when I practice *reiji hō,* I feel an almost magnetic pull, as if Reiki itself is moving my hands to the optimum place on the client's body or energy field. Although this is a dynamic and obvious response to my prayer, some people experience the effects of *reiji hō* in much more subtle ways. You may feel a sensation in your own body representative of where the origins of disharmony are in your client. You may see or hear where your hands should go. Or in lieu of any particular sign or pattern, you might just *know* where to place your hands.

Generally speaking, after placing your hands where Reiki guides you, it is likely that you will feel stronger *byōsen* there than in other parts of the body. While it may still take several minutes until you begin to recognize the sensations rising in your palms, stick with it until you can assess where the *byōsen* is and how strong it is. *Reiji hō* is not always an exact science; it will take practice for you to hone this intuitive art. If you are having difficulty working with *reiji hō,* try using the following method, *byōsen reikan hō,* or spend more time practicing the *gasshō* meditation and giving *yourself* Reiki.

Curiously, this technique of *reiji hō* nearly faded out of practice. Though still in use in the Usui Reiki Ryōhō Gakkai, it was not preserved in other systems of Reiki. Takata-sensei's diary records that she learned *reiji hō* from Hayashi-sensei in 1936, but she did not explicitly pass it on to her students. And although Hayashi taught *reiji hō* to Takata, he did not impart it to participants in his five-day seminars in Ishikawa; therefore, Yamaguchi Chiyoko never learned it. Currently, it is unknown whether Hayashi chose to omit *reiji hō* from the seminars in Ishikawa (where Yamaguchi and her family learned Reiki) because Hayashi had altered the format of his teachings when he traveled, or if Takata only learned it because she was his *uchideshi* and an advanced student.

1. Begin with a short *gasshō* meditation with your eyes closed.
2. When you feel Reiki flowing, place your hands, with palms still together, at the brow. Two variations exist: one with the fingertips pointed at the point between your eyebrows, and a second with the thumbs resting there instead.
3. With your hands at your brow, hold the intention to allow Reiki to guide your hands. The prayer I like to say is, "I ask my ego, attachment, and expectations to step aside so Reiki can be my guide."
4. Wait for a sign or indication (another translation of 示 is "indication" or "sign"). Whether this comes as a feeling, vision, symbol, or a desire to move your hands, place your hands accordingly.
5. Treat this location with Reiki, paying extra attention to the *byōsen* that you feel.

❖ *Byōsen Reikan Hō* 病腺靈感法

Byōsen reikan hō is one of the most popular Japanese techniques taught in Western branches of Reiki. It is most often called *byōsen scanning, and* the full name of this tool translates as "*byōsen* spiritual feeling method." The term *reikan* 靈感 usually translates as "inspiration," but in this case it also means "intuition." It is a fairly simple method for accessing your intuitive nature to find the location of *byōsen* in order to more effectively treat a client. This method and the one preceeding it serve as excellent tools for engaging your true self in the practice of Reiki, for they require the egoic self to take a back seat to the spirit.

The mechanics of *byōsen reikan hō* are very simple. After performing *gasshō,* the practitioner uses one or both hands to seek areas of depleted or imbalanced energy. *Byōsen* can be felt even at some distance from the body, so the hands are swept through the aura of the client in order to scan for target areas in need of Reiki. Additionally, the practitioner can adjust the height of his or her hand in order to treat various *layers* of the energy field. Since most illnesses originate in the aura or energy field, it may be possible to treat the *byōgen* (病元) without making physical contact with the client.

I have found that beginning practitioners often favor this method over the previous one because it appeals more to the conscious mind. Because it requires you to palpate the energy of your client, the mind understands why and where the hands are placed. If you find yourself having difficulty sensing *byōsen,* again, the remedy is to continue to practice; give yourself daily treatments and practice scanning yourself with this technique.

Byōsen scanning can be used at the start and end of a session as a means of tracking the progress of healing. You may find that patterns of disharmony, or *byōsen,* may shift location as a result of treatment. In addition to helping locate the most strategic position for treating clients, scanning enables the practitioner to ensure whether or not a treatment is ready to end. If the practitioner still feels locations that are emitting strong sensations, it may be necessary to continue treatment or to schedule another session with the same client for the near future.

1. Begin with a short *gasshō* meditation with your eyes closed.
2. When you feel Reiki flowing, place your hands, with palms still together, at the brow. Two variations exist: one with the fingertips pointed at the point between your eyebrows, and a second with the thumbs resting there instead.
3. As above, offer a prayer or statement of intent, such as "I ask that the consciousness of Reiki guide my hands on behalf of my client." By stating your intent to only be shown areas in need of Reiki, "you will not be distracted by the energy of a chakra or an organ or anything else unless that area needs Reiki."[7]
4. Using your most sensitive hand, or a combination of both hands, sweep slowly through the energy field of the client, beginning approximately one foot above his or her head. Move your hand(s) slowly and deliberately, noting any changes in the quality of the flow of Reiki. Wherever you feel *byōsen,* make a mental note. Remember that some of these energies may only be felt in the energy field of the client; it is okay to treat these areas above the body just as you would normally treat someone hands-on.

5. After scanning through the entire energy field at least once, locate the area with the most intense sensation of *byōsen* and treat that area first. Prioritizing higher levels of disharmony enables you to make the greatest amount of progress at the beginning of a session; some of the weaker *byōsen* that you feel are likely to stem from the stronger areas.

6. After a complete session, practice *byōsen reikan hō* in order to monitor the changes effected by Reiki.

❖ Chiryō 治療

The third and final pillar of *dento Reiki* is *chiryō*. *Chi* or 治 means "cure," "govern," or "rule." *Ryō* or 療 is "to cure or heal." Together, these kanji can be translated as "remedy," "healing method," "medical treatment," or "therapy." In Usui Reiki Ryōhō, *chiryō* is the (usually) hands-on application of Reiki energy in order to restore balance. In Japan, *chiryō* takes a variety of forms, with specific protocols recommended for certain conditions. Later branches of the Reiki family tree also use an abundance of different styles of treatment.

The simplest means of harnessing Reiki for healing is by laying on of hands. In Japanese, this act was a common healing tool, generally called *teate* and *tenohira*. These terms can be loosely translated as "hand placement" and "palm healing," respectively. As mentioned in chapter 2, many different styles of palm healing and other means of spiritual healing evolved in Japan, including other varieties of Reiki Ryōhō. Usui's method survives today and offers a simple, effective means of treating all manner of conditions.

Chiryō is the backbone of the Reiki system. I have met many people initiated into the system, including Masters/Teachers, who do not treat with Reiki regularly. Before we are anything else, we are students of the first degree *shoden,* which emphasizes simple, hands-on treatment above everything. The simplicity of Reiki Ryōhō is that we do not need any props or external tools; Reiki dwells within us always, so we can access it wherever we are by discreetly placing a palm on a convenient part of the body.

By engaging in hands-on healing, we are making space for healing. By committing our time and energy to healing ourselves or others, we are subconsciously sending the message that the recipient is worthy of wholeness. Gentle, noninvasive touch coupled with sincere presence and compassion are gifts that few people receive in today's world. Usui-sensei founded his method of Reiki Ryōhō in order to help bring us all back to our state of radiant health and an awareness of our true spiritual nature. In light of this, offering hands-on healing works in the same way that a guided meditation or spiritual journey helps others rediscover their inner wholeness.

Chiryō helps convert the intangible, mysterious qualities of Reiki into knowable, comprehensible forms. Without the hands-on practice, attaining *anshin ritsumei* would be an unlikely goal for most of us. However, holding this space for others—and ourselves—with compassionate abiding is a powerful catalyst for spiritual as well as physical healing. The mental and emotional patterns resolved by *gasshō meiso* and the spiritual patterns tapped into with *reiji hō* are brought into the physical through conventional hands-on healing. Together, the Three Pillars bring body, heart-mind (*kokoro*), and spirit into balance.

Usui left us a number of different ways to apply Reiki for healing. Many of these techniques and tools contain the word *chiryō* in their name, such as *heso chiryō* ("navel treatment") and *hanshin chiryō* ("half-body treatment"). He taught that after the first degree training, Reiki can be administered by placing the hands (*teate*), patting (*uchite chiryō hō*), stroking (*nadete chiryō hō*), pushing or applying pressure with the fingertips (*oshite chiryō hō*), and sending Reiki with the breath and eyes (*koki hō* and *gyōshi hō,* respectively). In many locations worldwide, practitioners are discouraged from any physical manipulations—such as patting, stroking, and pushing—unless they also have the proper training and licensure in massage or an equivalent technique.

In the remainder of the chapter you will find several ways of treating with Reiki, which originated in Japan. A number of other Reiki lineages teach similar techniques under other names. Before applying any of these methods during sessions with clients, practice them on yourself. Learn and master them so that you are comfortable with expanding the *chiryō* techniques beyond merely a laying on of hands.

❖ Koki Hō 呼氣法

In traditional Reiki Ryōhō, a particular family of techniques falls under the category of *kokyū hō* or 呼吸法, literally meaning "breathing techniques." Some of these are meditative tools, such as *joshin kokyū hō,* whereas others were meant to be applied during *chiryō,* such as this one. *Koki hō* is a means of harnessing the breath's natural flow of Reiki, and it translates as "exhalation method."

When practicing Reiki there are times when physical contact is not necessarily desired. In first aid scenarios, injuries such as cuts, scrapes, and especially burns can be too painful to be touched. Sanitary and hygienic concerns may also preclude hands-on healing, as can sensitive or private areas of the body. In these cases, sending Reiki with the breath can relieve discomfort and pain. When treating these scenarios, the practitioner generally uses a long exhalation with support from the diaphragm, as if playing a wind instrument.

In other circumstances, the breath can carry Reiki in a potentized pulse of energy that may be used to break up blockages. Whenever you sense stagnant or restricted energy flows, *koki hō* can be applied in order to break up the pattern causing disharmony. This echoes shamanic healing practices that also use the breath for healing. A rapid pulse of breath can transmit an intention from the practitioner as well, so it can be used to reprogram or rejuvenate an otherwise depleted area or incongruous energy. Because the forceful expulsion of air can sound startling to an otherwise relaxed client, be sure to let the client know that you will be making noise so as not to spoil his or her treatment.

Applying the breath in a short pulse can also be used to influence the cycle of *byōsen* during treatment. Once the cycle has reached its peak, the breath can be drawn in with the intention of breaking up the underlying cause, and it can be forcefully expelled on the target area. This typically brings the sensation of *byōsen* back to the beginning, which will reduce the overall treatment time because the practitioner no longer has to wait for the cycle to complete its falling action. On the next cycle, the *byōsen* will usually peak at a lower intensity, even if only slightly.

In the *okuden* training, three sacred symbols are introduced to students. These can also be combined with either method of *koki hō* in order to improve and specialize the power of healing with the breath.

Version One

1. Begin in *gasshō,* unless emergency situations make that difficult.
2. Focus your intention of concentrating Reiki energy into your breath.

3. Inhale deeply and hold the breath for a brief pause as you connect to the recipient or target area.

4. Exhale slowly through pursed lips, as if the air is a steady stream or thread being drawn through your lips. You can also use *gyōshi hō* with this method to enhance the efficacy.

5. Repeat as necessary.

Version Two

1. When treating with hands-on Reiki, find a specific area that feels stagnant, blocked, or disharmonious.

2. Focus your intention of concentrating Reiki with the breath. If you have a specific goal such as pain relief or rejuvenating the cells, for instance, you can connect to this specific energy, too.

3. Place the tip of your tongue on the roof of the mouth and inhale slowly and fully while concentrating on your intention.

4. Open your hands while maintaining contact with your client.

5. Pulse the breath onto the space outlined by your open hands; this should be a single, rapid breath.

6. Resume normal breathing while returning your hands to their position on the client. Continue to treat, paying close attention to *byōsen* in the target area.

7. Repeat as needed.

❖ Gyōshi Hō 凝視法

After the Great Kanto Earthquake in 1923, Usui Mikao is said to have treated thousands of people, many of them at the same time, and often using his eyes. The technique he taught for sending Reiki via the eyes is called *gyōshi hō,* which means "staring method." Usui noted that Reiki naturally flows through the hands, feet, eyes, and breath, so he instructed his students in various methods of controlling these natural outpourings of energy.

Much like *koki hō,* the use of *gyōshi hō* is helpful when physical contact is not possible or undesirable. Treating sensitive or off-limits areas can be accomplished through a gentle, unfocused gaze. *Gyōshi hō* is also ideal when the practitioner needs to treat more than one area simultaneously. The key is to connect to the flow of Reiki and consciously intend for it to be concentrated through the vision.

Gyōshi hō can also be used in nontraditional settings as a means of blessing or infusing an object or situation with Reiki. If you would like to charge your food with Reiki prior to eating it, the eyes can discreetly beam Reiki to your meal when you are in public, so as not to attract unwanted attention. You can send Reiki to your water, to gifts, to injured people you meet, and even to plants and animals in this way.

After training in *shoden,* first degree Reiki practitioners do not have all the tools to treat long distance, so a certain amount of proximity is required in order to enact *gyōshi hō.* Under normal conditions, you can use this technique from across the room or from other short distances. Its application includes treating the whole being at once. Indeed, I have found in my practice that it can be especially penetrating in cases of emotional disturbance and karma-related conditions.

When treating with your eyes, it is possible to feel *byōsen.* Although most students do not develop sensitivity immediately, experienced practitioners may become aware of a throbbing or tingling sensation in or behind the eyes during application of *gyōshi hō.* Don't be alarmed by these feelings; if they become uncomfortable, simply break eye contact for a few seconds before resuming treatment. Some practitioners also see symbols, colors, or flashes of insight while performing *gyōshi hō.* There is no need to interpret or cling to these images, but you may share them with your client if you choose.

1. Begin in *gasshō* position to connect to Reiki.
2. Close your eyes and intend for Reiki to flow through the eyes and into your client.
3. Open your eyes and gaze upon your client; employ an unfocused stare as if looking into or beyond the recipient. This can be used on a predetermined location or wherever your gaze feels drawn.
4. Breathe consciously and comfortably while sending Reiki; you may treat with your hands simultaneously.
5. When complete, gently relax your vision or close your eyes. Breathe in and out deeply, holding the intention to end the treatment.

❖ Heso Chiryō 臍治療

One technique not as well understood in the West is called *heso chiryō* or "treatment of the navel." In Japanese culture, the belly button is viewed as the seat of nurturing, given that it results from the scarring left by the umbilical cord that nourishes us as fetuses before birth. Chinese medicine considers this point as an important energy center, responsible for collecting our prenatal qi (氣, pronounced *ki* in Japanese). In a number of holistic modalities, it's also believed to be a recycling center and a doorway to accessing the internal organs for treatment.

The Japanese also believe that the navel has a powerful function in regulating temperature and overall health. When treating it via *heso chiryō,* Reiki serves to release excessive fire, or *ki,* in the body. This technique is therefore useful for conditions caused by physiological or pathological heat, or those that are influenced by fire according to Chinese medicine.

To target the umbilicus, the practitioner uses the middle finger of one hand. This is the fire finger, as described in the *gasshō* meditation. It therefore has a stronger output of Reiki energy than the other fingers, making it the best choice to be a concise point of focus. The tip of the middle finger is gently placed in or on the belly button, which can be done just as effectively through the client's clothing. Leave your hand in place until the *byōsen* has been resolved.

Bestselling Reiki author Frank Arjava Petter writes that this technique "is used in the treatment of cancer, fungal infections (internal as well as external candida for example), viral infections and fever."[8] It is a great technique for initiating systemic detoxification, treating the common cold and influenza, and regulating body temperature. *Heso chiryō* also helps moderate in cases where the internal organs are not functioning optimally; it may even offer success in jump-starting the metabolism. The Usui Reiki Ryōhō Gakkai "recommends healing on and around the navel at every opportunity since it builds up the immune system."[9] Friends and colleagues of mine have also found *heso chiryō* to be helpful in cases of hot flashes and tinnitus.

1. Bend the middle finger of either hand at the second joint and place the tip on the navel.

2. Apply even, gentle pressure and allow Reiki to flow. You will feel a rapid, perhaps erratic pulse separate from the flow of blood.

3. Monitor the rise and fall of *byōsen,* and continue to treat until it has stopped altogether.

❂ Tanden Chiryō 丹田治療 or Gedoku Hō 解毒法

The *tanden* in Japanese is synonymous to the *dantian* in Chinese; the term *tanden* refers to a series of centers or energy fields in our physical and spiritual anatomy. The three *tanden* are located at the brow, at the heart, and below the navel, and they are more or less analogous to the third eye, heart, and sacral chakras, respectively. *Tanden chiryō* focuses on the lower *tanden,* or *hara* (腹), which is located two to three finger-widths below the navel.

The *hara* is the seat of our life force, and it is also the home of Reiki in our bodies. After a *reiju* or initiation, Reiki flows from the universe into the crown and down to the *hara* before rising again and exiting through the palms of the hands. It is regarded as a critical area for treatment in Japanese (and Chinese) medical traditions; it is said to contain an energetic link to each of the major organs. The *hara* is also the seat of intuition, willpower, and vitality in Japanese culture, so treating this spot can promote positive mental and emotional adjustments, too.

Another technique, which is virtually identical in execution, is called *gedoku hō.* The kanji in the name of this technique mean to "solve" (解) and "poison" (毒); in combination they denote "detoxification" or "counteraction." Treating the lower *tanden* is a means of eliminating toxins from the body. Not limited to actual poison, *gedoku hō* can be used for food-borne illness and other digestive complaints, such as stomachache, constipation, and diarrhea.[10] After receiving this treatment, clients will frequently undergo the "healing reaction" that Takata described, wherein the eliminatory organs help dispose of toxins responsible for illness. Note that both techniques can easily be performed on oneself.

1. Place your dominant hand on the *hara,* just below the belly button, and your remaining hand directly opposite on the back of the body.

2. Treat until *byōsen* subsides or until the hands lift off on their own.

3. Optional: for *gedoku hō,* both practitioner and client can visualize the

toxins leaving via the eliminatory organs, including the intestines, kidneys, circulatory and lymphatic systems, and the skin.

In the next chapter we will delve into specifics of your practice, including how to build it and enhance it. You'll find practical advice that, when followed, will optimize the healing that you undertake, both for clients and for yourself.

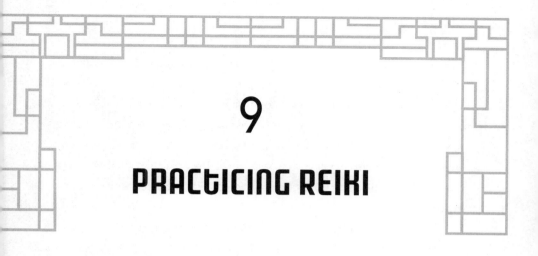

9

PRACTICING REIKI

THE MOST IMPORTANT ASPECT of Reiki Ryōhō is to make it a practice. To grow as a practitioner, one must commit time and energy to making Reiki a daily habit. Throughout this chapter we will explore some of the practical considerations of practicing Reiki, both personally and professionally.

PRACTICAL CONSIDERATIONS

Harnessing the Healing Power of Your Hands

Once you have received your initiation, Reiki energy flows easily and with little conscious direction. Applying Reiki can be as simple as placing your hands wherever you would like Reiki to flow. You may sense Reiki coursing through you spontaneously, especially shortly after *reiju*. It may also begin to flow whenever you are in proximity to a person or energy pattern that can benefit from this healing modality. Regular practice can help limit such energetic surprises, so be sure to give yourself Reiki regularly.

On a practical note, let's look at how to best use your hands during a Reiki session. The fingers should be held together for greater continuity of the energy. The effect is much like when you're swimming; if your fingers aren't together you would have difficulty propelling yourself forward. Your hands can be placed side by side or upon separate locations on the body according to the needs of a particular scenario.

If you prefer to treat according to prescribed hand positions, the hands are usually held in place for five to ten minutes in each location, unless your intuition or the cycles of *byōsen* indicate that you should stay longer or continue on. The hands can be moved one at a time from one location to the next so that you never lose contact with your client. Called Walking the Hands, this practice ensures that the recipient is continuously energized by Reiki.

Reiki projected from the whole hand covers wide areas with a gentle wave of Reiki that helps saturate a given area. For wider target areas, it's best that your hands are positioned together. This makes for an even, diffuse dose of Reiki energy. When a more deeply penetrating effect is necessary, the hands can be stacked one on top of the other; this can be used to permeate the physical body and heal a specific organ or injured area. This is an especially loving gesture when applied over your heart or the heart of a client.

The fingertips can be used to focus the energy of Reiki for more specific or delicate areas. Much like in *heso chiryō,* a single finger can be placed over small points in order to treat them with Reiki. The index or middle finger is preferable, but a combination of fingers can be used for many areas, such as treating a specific vertebra, the ears, the eyes, the lymph nodes, or the toes. When more power and focus are required, all of the fingers may be shaped into a cone, which directs Reiki through the tips of the fingers into a powerful, laser-like beam. This method can be used to pinpoint small or sensitive locations, including teeth, lymph glands, eyes, ear canals, the brain stem, or points along the meridians.

In locations that are hard to reach, such as the kidneys, you can choose to treat yourself with the backs of your hands rather than the palms. The energy centers responsible for dispensing Reiki are chakras or vortexes of energy in your hands. These energy centers extend as funnels of energy in two directions (from both the palms and the backs of your hands). This can help you treat some places on the back for greater lengths of time in order to clear away persistent *byōsen.*

Again, Reiki may be practiced with or without physical contact.

The hands may be placed directly on the area being treated, or they can be held two to three inches above it. Reiki flows first into the energy field of the recipient this way, and it will then begin to saturate the cells of the physical body just below where the hands are held. Hands-off treatments can be used in situations where touch is undesirable, such as extremely painful areas, or where it is unethical to touch, such as over the private areas of your clients' anatomy. In regions where touch is prohibited without proper licensure (e.g., a massage therapy license or a nursing certificate), Reiki can be employed without touch. It also easily penetrates clothing, sheets, and blankets, so clients have no need to disrobe.

Preparing an Environment for Healing

Reiki is simple and can be effectively administered in virtually any location. However, if you prefer to take your healing into the professional arena, certain factors of your environment should be considered. Cleanliness and hygiene are important. The space itself can become an extension of your Reiki practice by providing a nurturing container in which deep relaxation and surrender to the healing process may ensue.

Choose soft lighting, bearing in mind that some clients may prefer natural light while others may prefer a dimmer setting. Light, peaceful colors and decor are more appropriate than neons and dark shades. Keep the space free of clutter, and select decor that supports healing, such as images of Usui-sensei, spiritual art, crystals, sacred statues, and other tools that will anchor the practice of Reiki Ryōhō. You may also choose to create a healing altar.

Essential oils, candles, and incense are lovely additions to your healing space, but remember that not every client can tolerate their scents, so it would be wise to burn them only with your clients' permission. Soothing music is also a great tool, but be sure to give your clients the option of choosing from your favorite healing sounds or to enjoy noble silence.

Offer your clients a comfortable place to lie down, such as a massage table, or use seating that enables you to treat whichever areas are pertinent. Some people prefer to position themselves either faceup or facedown; remember that you can treat the body from either side because Reiki will flow wherever it is most needed. If possible, coordinate with your client's position so that you can most easily treat his or her specific concerns.

Wherever you offer Reiki sessions, make that space as comfortable and inviting as possible. If you practice out of your home, remove anything distracting or unkempt. Turn off phones, tablets, or other distractions so that you can be fully and compassionately present for whoever is receiving Reiki. You can even learn to treat yourself this way! Be mindful of the energy in your room before and after treatment. You may cleanse or clear the space by chanting the Five Principles as in *gokai sansho,* or you may use other tools to do so. This is especially needed after a session in which a client may have released deleterious energy patterns in the course of receiving Reiki.

Explaining Reiki to Others

As we practice with greater frequency, we will eventually have opportunities to share Reiki with people who are unfamiliar with what it is. In these cases, we are tasked with describing something as esoteric and magical as Reiki in terms that are accessible to outsiders. While a simple translation of the term *Reiki* as "universal life force" may be adequate in many cases, it will not always suffice. This is where we learn to take examples from our own experiences with Reiki and allow it to teach us how to introduce others to Reiki Ryōhō.

I don't usually have a single go-to response when someone asks me about Reiki. I find that it's easy to describe it as a healing system that stems from early twentieth-century Japan, with documented benefits including stress reduction and pain management. However, describing the *system* and the *energy* are two very different things. For many people who are spiritually inclined, Reiki can be translated as a spiritually guided form of ki or qi; it can also be described as *soul energy, God power,* or *unconditional love.*

Explaining what Reiki is and how it works can put prospective clients at ease. As Reiki practitioners, we can be ambassadors for this system of natural healing. However, we must learn to use tact and sensibility when we describe its effects, and we must support our claims with illustrations of times it has worked in our own lives.

Intention and Consent

One minor point of contention among Reiki practitioners is the subject of setting an intention when we practice Reiki. Reiki itself, as a conscious and spiritual energy, needs no guidance or instructions from either sender or receiver. However, learning how to train the mind is an important aspect of Reiki Ryōhō. Although healing in any modality is certainly an intentional, conscious process, the manner in which we direct our intent can influence the result.

Whether we are practicing on ourselves or treating others, intent can change the game entirely. As we develop our Reiki triggers, we are clearly intending to connect to Reiki to heal the recipient. However, we cannot guide Reiki to cure or heal any particular condition; the divine intelligence overseeing the healing process has its own agenda according to the physical, psychological, karmic, and spiritual path of the person being treated. Although Reiki can often induce miraculous healing, it only does so under the right circumstances.

Thus, as practitioners, we harness the power of our intention by choosing to be the conduit for healing, not by intending what the outcome of healing is supposed to be. Reiki is a lesson in surrender, for both the recipient *and* the practitioner. The client is surrendering by being totally relaxed and open to whatever tools the practitioner employs, and the Reiki facilitator is surrendering his or her control of the situation to the Divine, so that Reiki can flow wherever and however is best for all parties. And although we cannot guarantee a specific result from Reiki, certain outcomes are so likely as to be almost guaranteed. These include relaxation, rejuvenation, enhanced sleep, and reduced pain.

The best intentions to set revolve around compassion, love, and surrender. You cannot make Reiki change its course any more than you can change the direction of the Earth's movement around the sun. Instead, make yourself an empty vessel so that more and more Reiki can flow through you and be made available to whoever is receiving your healing touch. Reiki will do all the work so that your client (and you!) can transform accordingly.

The issue of consent falls under similar jurisdiction, as Reiki is ultimately only able to work according to the highest needs of the recipient. Most Western practitioners cite rules or guidelines that Reiki should only ever be given when the recipient asks for or consents to treatment specifically. However, looking into original Japanese documents may shed some light on this question.

The Usui Reiki Ryōhō Gakkai issues a handbook to its students and practitioners titled the *Reiki Ryōhō Hikkei* (靈氣癒法必携, Reiki Healing Method Manual), which contains a series of questions and answers provided by Usui-sensei himself. When asked if one needs to believe in Reiki Ryōhō for results to be achieved, he responds thus: "No, unlike psychological therapy, hypnotism, and other mental healing modalities, no consent nor esteem is required, for not a single suggestion is given. Moreover, it matters little whether you may doubt, avoid, and deny that. For instance, there is a positive effect on those who lack consciousness, such as infants and/or seriously ill patients. Barely one out of ten people trust and esteem any art of healing before they experience it the first time. Most people come to trust suddenly after having received treatment once and acknowledged its effect."[1] Usui makes it clear that the recipient is not required to believe in, trust, or even ask for treatment with Reiki in order for it to be effective.

From a Japanese perspective, the greater good often emerges as being more important than the individual good. In the case of healing and spiritual awakening, those people who are empowered to offer healing are encouraged to do so as widely as possible. To heal any one person's illness is to heal the world's total illness, even if only a little. If we choose to look at it from another perspective, the higher self is truly the aspect of one's self that elects to accept or deny healing. Since Reiki is the action of unconditional love and compassion, there is very little likelihood that *anyone's* higher self would reject unconditional love.

Just because we can send healing without consent does not always make it the best option. The main reason that so many teachers stress a need for consent is because it empowers the client to be involved in his or her own healing. By consciously electing to seek help in any form, including Reiki, we are putting our energy into making ourselves well again. Because of this, when someone actively chooses to receive Reiki, they feel liberated from the limiting patterns of pain, disease, and disharmony.

Duration and Frequency

When treating any condition, it is vital to remember that Reiki is not usually going to solve a problem overnight. In chronic cases especially, we need to be realistic about therapeutic outcomes. We can encourage clients with long-term conditions to stay the course of treatment until the concern is totally resolved or managed, which varies from one example to another. The most important thing to remember is that when we treat, we can use *byōsen* as an indicator that reveals how the healing progresses.

A standard treatment usually lasts an hour or more. If you are treating with a standardized set of hand positions, spend five to ten minutes in each location unless a strong sensation of *byōsen* invites you to remain in one locus for a longer amount of time. Chronic and critical illness or injury generally have more pervasive and more intense levels of *byōsen*, such as the strong throbbing (*hibiki*) or pain/discomfort (*itami*) mentioned earlier. *Byōsen* such as these will require a longer treatment time.

From one treatment to the next, the levels of *byōsen* often fluctuate. Because life does not stop after a Reiki session, your client's *byōsen* are likely to change. Even if the sensation has diminished significantly in one session, it will likely exhibit strong levels again on the client's next visit. Regular and frequent treatments will make lasting changes over time.

For acute conditions, daily treatment over the course of a few days to a week will usually resolve illness and pain. A common cold or flu can often be mitigated if treated several times a day at the onset of the earliest symptoms. When self-treating, this can be as simple as placing a free hand on the afflicted area whenever you have time to do so.

When treating, remember that there is no such thing as overdosing on Reiki. It never causes harm, never depletes, has no contraindication, and is always a joy to give and receive. You also cannot give "too little" Reiki, as any Reiki is better than none. Over time you will gain experience to help you understand the progression of both illness and healing, so that you may coach your clients and yourself on the best treatment protocol for all involved parties.

Documentation and Money

When beginning your Reiki practice, it's a great habit to start taking notes on each of your treatments. Even if you have no intention of practicing professionally, good notes can help you learn from one treatment to the next. You can incorporate this aspect of practice into each session, so that you're well informed about the condition(s) of your clients and can watch their progress with Reiki.

A simple client information form or treatment documentation form should include your client's basic personal information and the nature of their concerns and overall health. It should also have room to note the locations on the body that you have treated. Take time to include each of the methods you've used and what the sensations of *byōsen* were. If you feel inspired, you can graph the overall pattern of the *byōsen* sensations, which will enable you to look for commonalities among different conditions and people.

If you are practicing for money, bear in mind what the rules and regulations of your state, province, and country may be. In some locations there are no requirements for practicing Reiki professionally, while other regions may require a massage license or another license. In some places ordained ministers may also practice Reiki and other healing modalities as part of their ministry with no additional licensure required; you can obtain legal ordination online for little or no cost if this is an option you would like to pursue. Do your research before charging money in exchange for Reiki treatments. The use of client release forms, examples of which can be found online, are also a good practice to maintain, as they may protect you from future upsets.

On the topic of money, in a professional setting many Reiki practitioners will charge rates comparable to the current cost of a massage or other bodywork session. This is very reasonable, so be sure to compare the prices you would like to set with the prices other practices are charging. The more you practice and the more tools you can master, the higher the compensation you may choose to ask for in return for your sessions.

Historically, Reiki training was very expensive, although, that said, it is also true that treatments were often free. Western lineages stemming from Usui Shiki Ryōhō often cite Takata's lesson about an energy exchange, wherein a session will only be appreciated and integrated if paid for. However, anecdotal evidence suggests that in the early days of *dento Reiki* in Japan, sessions were compensated for with whatever a client had; a farmer might bring rice, while a fisherman might trade fish. In emergency situations, Reiki was freely offered, such as when Usui treated thousands of people after the Great Kanto Earthquake of 1923.

FACETS OF A REIKI TREATMENT

Below I will outline the various stages of a full Reiki session. Bear in mind that not each and every one of these steps may be necessary or even possible. In emergency situations, it is generally impossible to explain Reiki and have the recipient fill out a client information form. Reiki is highly adaptable, so you can modify the overall flow of your practice to any scenario you might encounter. Some of the following steps will refer to the Japanese Reiki Techniques, whereas others will make use of more recent tools added to the system, which are detailed in chapter 12. The choice is yours as to which tools you will apply in your sessions.

Practice common sense and good hygiene when offering Reiki to others. Always have a clean space, freshly washed hands, and pillows or blankets available. You can use spare pillows to prop up your own arms and hands so they don't tire during treatments, and to prevent yourself from placing too much weight on your client's body. If someone's condition is severe, or if they have a communicable disease, always encourage them to visit their primary health care provider. Remember that Reiki complements conventional medicine; it does not replace it.

Introduction and Anamnesis

When meeting a client for the first time, introduce yourself warmly and take the time to get to know him or her on a cursory level. This may be your client's first experience with complementary or integrative healing practices, so you may need to explain what Reiki is and how it works. Afterward, you can complete a client intake form or jot down some notes about what he or she wishes to have treated. Keep your notes in an accessible location so that you can keep track of the session.

During this step you can decide on the course of treatment. For general maintenance or unknown conditions, you can use a prescribed set of hand positions, or you may simply want to wait and see where scanning or *reiji hō* will lead you. For known disorders or injuries, you can investigate to find the most efficient way of treating. Remember to focus on the *byōgen,* or "origin of illness," which may or may not be directly related to the symptoms.

Help your client find his or her own best state of relaxation. Your client will be lying down or seated for the treatment in most instances, so give him or her a moment or two to unwind after climbing onto the table. You may offer a brief guided visualization or simply encourage your client to breathe deeply and let go of tension wherever he or she feels it in the body.

Connecting to Reiki

Once the recipient is relaxed, spend a moment in *gasshō* as you connect to Reiki. You may recite the *gokai* or use your favorite prayer or affirmation as you do so. I like to include a request that Reiki work on behalf of the recipient's highest path. Once you feel Reiki energy flowing within and through you, use *kenyoku hō* or the Reiki Shower to cleanse and charge your entire energy field. You can also hold your hands in front of you (or to each side) with your palms facing inward in order to beam Reiki to your own center as means of empowering you before treating others.

Beaming Reiki

With Reiki-charged hands, step away from your client and beam the energy from several feet away. This enables you to treat your client's entire energy field as a whole. This simple step takes only minutes but is gently nourishing and supportive for the recipient. Beaming healing vibrations in this way also helps establish an energetic rapport, thereby sensitizing you and attuning you to the recipient's energy field; afterward, in the next step, you are more likely to get results. Optionally you might consider using the Opening Spiral (see page 212).

Byōsen Reikan or Reiji Hō

Accessing your intuition can help you streamline your treatment by leading you to the areas of strongest *byōsen*. Employ either *reiji hō* or *byōsen reikan hō* to help locate the most strategic locations for treatment. Sometimes these areas will be aligned with the symptoms, whereas in other examples the origin may be an imbalance seemingly unrelated to the symptoms.

Whichever method you choose should play to your strengths. If you are good at picking up subtle sensations, use the scanning method. On the other hand, if you trust your instincts or have good visualization skills, try *reiji hō* instead. It helps to practice these techniques frequently on yourself or your loved ones in order to polish them for use with others.

Hands-On Treatment

This stage reflects where the majority of your time and energy will be spent. The third pillar of Reiki is treatment (*chiryō*), and this is where you are able to perfect it. After isolating the area(s) in greatest need of Reiki, use hands-on or hands-off methods according to the needs and preferences of your client. At this stage you may follow your treatment guidelines for set hand positions (see chapter 11) or proceed by simply treating where you find *byōsen*.

Chiryō can take many forms, making it highly adaptable to each individual's unique conditions. You can employ any of the Japanese Reiki Techniques or some of the newer tools from Western styles of Reiki. Try gazing with Reiki (*gyōshi hō*) or sending it with the breath (*koki hō*). Keep track of the sensations of *byōsen* so that you may record them afterward. Having a clock or a timer nearby is a useful practice as well, for it ensures adherence to your schedule and allows you to time the rise and fall of each cycle of *byōsen*.

Closing Procedures

Once treatment is complete, take a few moments to wrap things up. Gently sweeping through the client's energy field may help eliminate stray patterns of disharmony. Visualize this acting like the Reiki Shower, wherein Reiki envelops the aura of your client and helps cleanse it of the patterns being released. Use one or two sweeps down each side and over the center of the client's body.

Next, you may choose to do one final pass of *byōsen reikan hō* to check the status of your client's healing process. Note where you have felt *byōsen* so that you can monitor these locations on his or her next visit. Scanning before and after treatment helps verify the progress overall and will guide you to locate the origins of conditions more accurately.

Finally, hold your hands over the *hara* (near the navel) of your client and silently pray or intend for the healing to be sealed. This serves to demarcate the end of the treatment session, disconnect your awareness from your client's energy field, and help maintain the positive effects of Reiki in your client's life. A simple affirmation that you can repeat is, "This healing is sealed with unconditional love." You may also want to incorporate the Closing Spiral (see page 212) into your ending procedures.

Cleansing

After closing the session, a brief cleansing is ideal. Using *kenyoku hō* or the Reiki Shower (or another cleansing technique or tool) helps you maintain good spiritual hygiene. You should physically wash your hands, especially before treating another client. It can be helpful to light a candle or burn incense or sage, too, so long as it will not disturb your client. Repeating the *gokai* can also be used to cleanse the space between sessions, and you can perform *jaki kiri jōka hō* (see page 264) to cleanse your massage table or any other implements you may have used in the session. Ensure that your own well-being and the energy of your healing space are taken care of before, during, and after each and every treatment.

Following Up

After a Reiki treatment, gently bring your client back to normal waking consciousness. Many people doze off or enter a state of deep relaxation or contemplation. A gentle tap or rub on the shoulder will usually suffice. Ask him or her to sit up with caution, allowing your client time to integrate the experience of receiving Reiki at his or her own pace. I always offer a fresh glass of water after treatment (however, bear in mind that as Reiki practitioners we cannot make this sound as if it is a medical recommendation).

After treatment you may share with your client any intuitive messages, symbols, or perceptions you may have received during the session. Perhaps you would like to discuss the sensations you may have felt from his or her *byōsen*. However, again, remember that unless you are medically trained and licensed, you may *not* use this as a diagnosis. Ask your client if he or she would like to share their experience of receiving Reiki, making note of any physical or subtle feelings or messages they received.

Encourage your clients to be gentle with themselves after a Reiki treatment, inviting them to spend time in nature, to be mindful, and to drink more water. You may also schedule a follow-up session or a series of sessions as a treatment protocol to ensure that any preexisting conditions are completely resolved or managed to the best of the client's ability. Of course, if there is any severe *byōsen* or cautionary intuitive impression, you can tactfully invite a client to consult with a primary health care provider.

WHEN REIKI DOESN'T WORK

The more we familiarize ourselves with treating conditions with Reiki, the more miracles we will experience. I have seen burns disappear within seconds and choking overcome without the administration of the Heimlich maneuver, watched chronic pain dissolve, and seen infectious and chronic diseases reverse themselves in short amounts of time. In spite of the mounting evidence that Reiki can, and often will, amaze us, there are times when it appears as if Reiki cannot help or cure some conditions.

The bottom line is that not every illness can be resolved. There will be times when you cannot save a life or stop disease in its tracks. When these events occur, be mindful of what Reiki is offering under these circumstances. Reiki is proven to provide relaxation, and studies are showing its efficacy in alleviating pain and combating illnesses such as cancer and other chronic diseases. Although we may not always see measurable effects with Reiki, it is always working for the highest order of both practitioner and recipient.

In cases where critical and terminal illnesses are being treated with Reiki, it may be that its only results are deep relaxation. This sense of peace can help prepare individuals with terminal illness for their transitions. Reiki is the energy of love and compassion, and offering it to people in need always helps, even if only in subtle ways. Whenever Reiki is practiced responsibly, it is a pleasant adjunct to allopathic medicine, and it may support the restorative and palliative efforts of conventional treatments.

There are many reasons why treatment with Reiki Ryōhō may not result in a complete recovery. Some illnesses are, quite simply, terminal ones. Independent of a client's desire to get well again, there will be times when Reiki is unable to change the prognosis. In these cases Reiki energy offers itself in loving service no matter the outcome. Reiki might simply remind people that love and compassion still exist in the world, even if it does nothing to alter the course of a specific illness or injury. In cases such as these, practitioners should not equate "losses" or a lack of improvement with failure. On the contrary, scenarios like these are often beautiful experiences for both practitioner and recipient alike as the soul readies itself to cross over.

Reiki cannot be relied upon as the only tool for making everyone well. We all interact with sickness, medicine, and energy differently. Because of this, Reiki will not always be the right tool or the *only* tool for every client. Exercise tact and be as ethical as you can when treating a patient with a critical illness. And remember that Reiki never causes harm, so we can always envelop clients and loved ones in its compassionate, soothing energy.

10

HAND POSITIONS FOR SELF-TREATMENT

MRS. TAKATA TAUGHT A STANDARDIZED treatment in her *shoden* classes as a means of simplifying and codifying protocols. This framework serves to ensure that Reiki is given to all major parts of the body, targeting major organs, large joints, and the various energy centers. Treating in this way helps the beginning student build confidence, apply Reiki wherever *byōsen* usually lurks, and add structure to an otherwise formless and intuitive art.

When I first learned Reiki, our teacher provided manuals with detailed illustrations of protocols for treating ourselves and others; our very first sessions were run according to these instructions. Thereafter, our teacher helped us tap into our inner guidance in order to practice Reiki Ryōhō more intuitively. Since then I have rarely utilized a rigid structure, but in spite of my preference for a less structured approach, I've found that adding a pattern of hand positions makes Reiki easy to learn for practitioners who are not yet ready to rely upon their intuition.

Takata-sensei admonished her students to follow the guidance of their hands; if it felt as though we should stay longer in a particular location or stray from the standard treatment, then surely Reiki would be guiding that impression. A standardized treatment plan simply helps build a platform of practicing Reiki by staying in the flow of the energy. Remember, Reiki is life force that is simultaneously spiritual, universal, intelligent, and effective. It walks us into wholeness through its action of awakening the true self.

I have adapted the following hand positions from Takata's teachings, which she called the Foundation Treatment. Many variations on the standard hand positions exist, so I selected the most commonly recommended ones from historical sources and tempered them with my own experience. Additionally, I've added a few extra locations not normally included in Takata's twelve standard positions. These are optional, though treating the lower extremities is generally extremely balancing and leaves one feeling very grounded after treatment.

Experiment with the different methods of treatment as you gain proficiency with Reiki. In the standard treatment, each position is usually treated for five to ten minutes; listen to your intuition if you feel it's beneficial to deviate from the timing or location of each place. It's imperative to note that it's always more productive to treat *byōsen* than to insist upon following a standard schedule of hand positions.

The Foundation Treatment does not cover every part of the body. Thus, if illness or injury impacts another location, use your judgment and add any afflicted area to your treatment plan. Emergency situations frequently invite practitioners to treat outside the following positions.

FOUNDATION FOR SELF-TREATMENT

Please note that dotted lines in the following diagrams represent where the hands should be placed to treat the back of the body; contiguous lines represent where the hands should be placed to treat the front of the body or the sides of the body.

1. Place the hands gently over the eyes, with the fingertips approximately at the hairline. Position 1 treats the eyes, sinuses, mouth, and brain.

2. The hands cover the sides of the head. Usually the palms cover the ears, but the hands may instead slide upward so that the fingertips touch at the crown. Position 2 offers Reiki to the ears, inner ears, mandibular joints, and brain.

3. Place the hands together at the back of the skull. The heels of your hands will cradle the spot where the skull and vertebrae meet, which is called the Mouth of God in Chinese medicine. This position supports the health of all the organs of the head, the nervous system, and the cervical vertebrae. It can be especially effective for headaches.

4. The hands come together over the throat; alternatively, place one hand at the throat and one over the thymus (upper chest). Position 4 saturates the throat, lymph glands, thymus, trachea and esophagus, thyroid, jaw, and mouth with Reiki energy.

5. Place the hands over the sternum, covering as much of the heart and lungs as possible. You may also treat each side of the rib cage as a separate position. Position 5 gives Reiki to the heart, lungs, thymus, and other organs of the upper chest. This is a very relaxing way to give Reiki before falling asleep at night.

6. Move the hands to your abdomen, spanning the area from the uppermost abdomen where the stomach lies to the lower part of your midsection so that your intestines are also treated. It is also possible to treat the midsection separately, as if partitioning the torso into quadrants. Position 6 nourishes the stomach, liver, intestines, diaphragm, and gallbladder with Reiki.

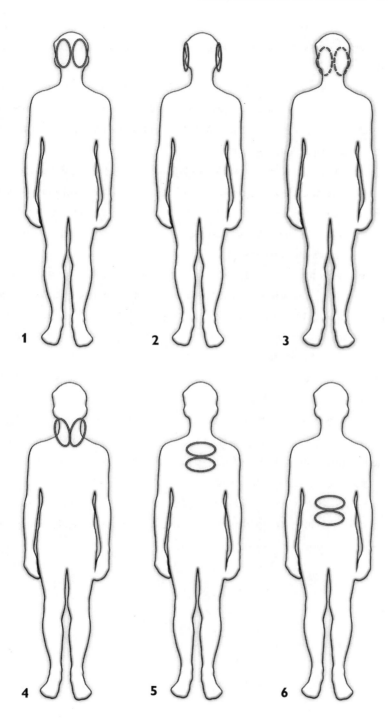

7. Treat the sides of the abdomen. This hand position offers Reiki to the liver, large intestine, and spleen, as well as to the muscles of the midsection.

8. The hands line up to treat the lowest portion of the abdomen. From this position, the intestines, appendix, and *hara* or lower *tanden* are treated. Treating the *hara* is enlivening and rejuvenating—it helps restore one's personal power and life force.

9. Slant the hands downward and slightly lower (than the previous position). From here, the pelvic floor, hips, and muscles of the groin are treated. The sex organs also receive Reiki as the energy saturates the cells and gradually moves to the surrounding area. The lymph nodes nearby are the recipients of Reiki as well.

10. Place the hands on or between the shoulder blades. It may be more comfortable for some practitioners to cross their arms (holding them higher up, by the neck) to maintain this position for the full length of treatment. There is usually a fairly strong emanation from the *byōsen* stored here, which often persists due to the difficulty of self-treatment. The joints of the neck, shoulders, and upper back also benefit from this position.

11. Place the hands over the kidneys; if necessary, close your hands and place the back of your fists against the kidneys. Treating this location offers Reiki to the adrenals, pancreas, spleen, the muscles of the back and, of course, to the kidneys themselves.

12. Move the hands to the lower back so that the fingertips meet at the coccyx. Healing is shared with the base of the spine, hips, pelvic bowl, rectum, glutes, and lower back.

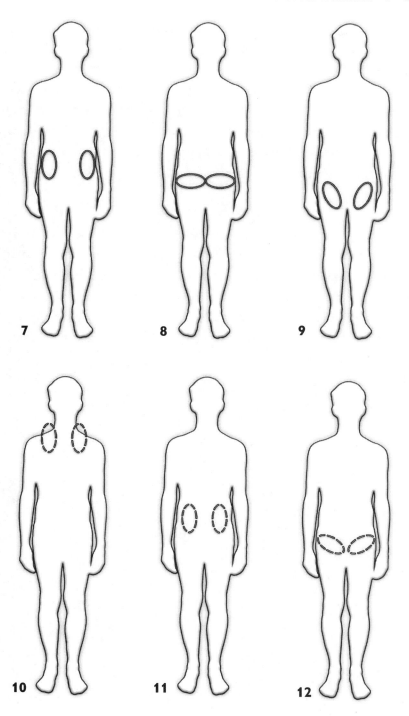

13. Treat the knees. They can be treated together or one at a time, with the hands cradling each knee separately.

14. Treat the feet, either together or separately. They are easy to reach in bed or when you're seated cross-legged. Try beaming Reiki to your feet if you can't easily place your hands on them. According to reflexology, the feet mirror the entire body, so they help disperse healing to the whole system. Treating them last also ensures that you're grounded and fully embodied after a Reiki session.

Optional Positions

15. Place one hand at the brow and one over the back of the head. Treating this combination envelops the brain with Reiki energy. It helps calm an overactive mind and treats headache, insomnia, and congestion.

16. One hand on the brow and one hand at the heart help instill harmony between mental and emotional energies. This combination helps the practitioner achieve the heart-mind unity referred to by the term *kokoro,* or 心 in Japanese.

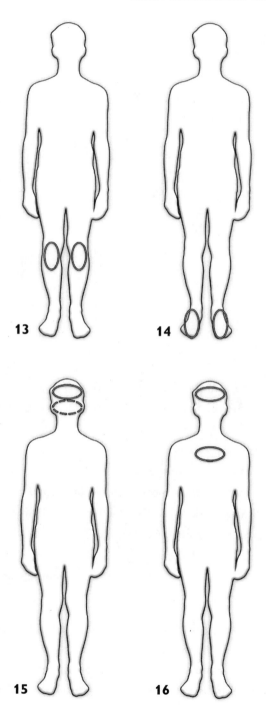

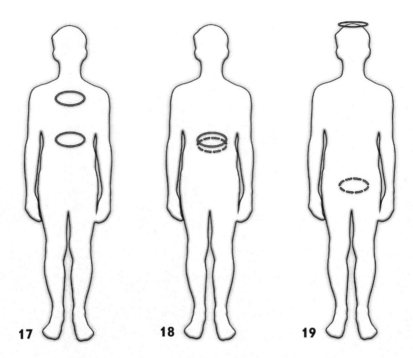

17.   Place one hand at the heart and one over the solar plexus. The lungs, heart, and thymus benefit, as do the stomach and diaphragm. This is one of the most calming hand positions for self-treatment, and it's especially effective in treating anxiety, stress, and panic.

18.   One hand rests at the stomach, while the other treats the opposite side of the body, though slightly lower. This combination targets the gastrointestinal system, making it effective for digestive complaints such as upset stomach, diarrhea, bloating, and constipation.

19.   Place one hand at the crown and one over the base of the spine on the back of the body. This is effective for a quick tune-up, and it leaves one feeling refreshed, alert, and grounded.

The next chapter will cover hand positions for treating others. As you will see, many of these are the same as those articulated in this chapter. We discuss them again before moving on to some new exercises that will benefit those you are seeking to heal with the wonderful practice of Reiki.

11

HAND POSITIONS FOR TREATING OTHERS

THE BASIC POSITIONS FOR TREATING OTHERS are fundamentally similar to those for self-treatment, which includes treating both the front and the back of the body. It should be noted that in some cases, the individual you are treating may be unable to lie either faceup or facedown on your table (due to their physical limitations) or they may simply fall asleep during a treatment. There is no great need to awaken them; merely treat whatever you can reach. Reiki will saturate each area of the body beneath the hands and gradually spread to areas beyond your reach.

Using a standard set of hand positions is not usually a replacement for seeking out and targeting *byōsen*. In many cases, the stronger levels of *byōsen* such as *hibiki* and *itami* simply cannot be detected within the five minutes usually allotted for the Foundation Treatment. However, regular practice in any form or style will sensitize the hands over time. If you're unfamiliar with *byōsen* or are still developing the sensitivity and intuition needed to help you locate areas of disharmony, use the foundation positions as a means of providing a thorough and effective treatment.

The following hand positions, like those in the previous chapter, are largely inspired by Hawayo Takata and the teachings of her lineage.

197

They can be adapted to suit the needs of a particular individual and they make an excellent treatment for individuals seeking the maintenance of good health.

FOUNDATION TREATMENT FOR OTHERS

Please note that dotted lines in the following diagrams represent where the hands should be placed to treat the back of the body; contiguous lines represent where the hands should be placed to treat the front of the body or the sides of the body.

1. Place the hands gently over the eyes, with the heel of your palms approximately at the hairline. The first position treats the eyes, sinuses, mouth, and brain.
2. The hands cover the sides of the head. Usually the ears are covered, but the hands may instead slide upward so that the palms nearly touch at the crown. Position 2 offers Reiki to the ears, inner ears, mandibular joints, and brain.
3. Place the hands together at the back of the skull by gently rocking the head to one side and sliding the first hand beneath it and repeating in the opposite direction to place the second hand. The fingertips rest at the spot where the skull and vertebrae meet, called the Mouth of God in Chinese medicine. This position supports the health of all the organs of the head, the nervous system, and the cervical vertebrae. It can be especially effective for headaches.
4. The hands come together over the throat; alternatively, place one hand at the throat and one over the thymus (upper chest). Many people are uncomfortable having their throat or neck touched for prolonged periods of time; check in with your client and adjust as needed. You may treat hands-off by hovering just above the throat. Position 4 saturates the throat, lymph glands, thymus, trachea and esophagus, thyroid, jaw, and mouth with Reiki energy.

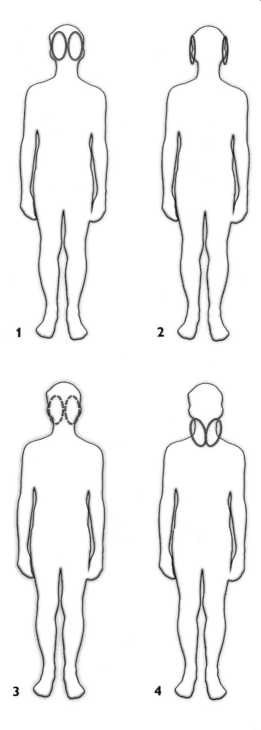

5. Place the hands over the sternum in a *T*-shaped formation. You may also treat each side of the rib cage as a separate position. Position 5 gives Reiki to the heart, lungs, thymus, and other organs of the upper chest. You might expect to hear a deep sigh of relaxation from your client if you haven't already.

6. Align the hands as if they form a band across your client's solar plexus. Position 6 centers on the diaphragm, stomach, liver, gallbladder, and spleen.

7. Move the hands approximately one hand-width lower to treat the lower part of the liver, large intestine, and spleen, as well as the muscles of the midsection.

8. The hands move to treat the lowest portion of the abdomen. From this position, the intestines, appendix, and *hara* or lower *tanden* are treated. The uterus or prostate is also reached from this position.

9. Slant the hands downward and slightly lower than the previous position so that they form a *V*. From here, the pelvic floor, hips, and muscles of the groin are treated. The sex organs also receive Reiki as the energy saturates the cells and gradually moves to the surrounding area. The lymph nodes nearby receive Reiki as well. (Ensure that your hands are in neutral territory so that no one's trust or comfort level is breached accidentally.)

10. Treat the thighs, either together or separately. There is a lot of muscle in the upper portion of the legs and into the hips, and treating here can alleviate long-standing tension.

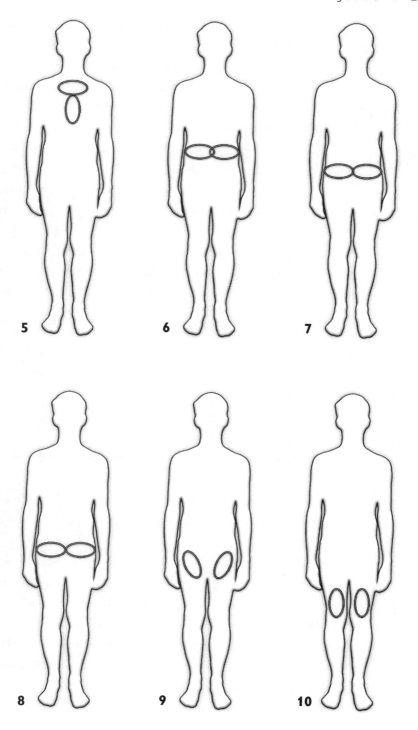

11. Treat the knees. They can be treated together or one at a time, with the hands cradling each one from the top and bottom. The knees often overcompensate for injuries or pain in the lower back, hips, ankles, and feet. Many people may even be unaware of the additional stress placed on one or both knees. If you are only treating the front of the body, skip ahead to position 18; otherwise, continue to position 12.

12. With your client facedown, place your hands on the shoulder blades. This is a benign place for toxins to be stored at the physical level, and as a result, most people emanate strong *byōsen* here. Utilizing this position, Reiki will nourish the shoulders, underarm lymph nodes, neck, and upper back.

13. The hands can be held in a straight line to treat the upper back. Or conversely, for conditions with an emotional cause, the hands can be placed side by side or one on top of the other over the back of the heart instead.

14. Place the hands over the middle of the back, maintaining the same alignment as positions 12 and 13. In addition to the muscles of the back and the spine itself, this position treats the stomach, liver, gallbladder, and spleen from the reverse side of the body.

15. The hands move to the kidneys, also treating the adrenals, pancreas, spleen, and muscles of the back.

16. Move the hands down to the lower back. This position enables you to treat the upper part of the pelvis and the lower spine.

17. Treat the hips and coccyx, using either a *T*-shaped or a *V*-shaped hand position. This treats the coccyx, hips, sacrum, prostate (in men), intestines, appendix, rectum, and glutes.

18. The feet may be treated simultaneously—with the hands placed wherever it's most comfortable for the practitioner—or the feet may be treated individually one after the other, cradling the top and bottom of each foot with both hands. As we have established, all of the parts of the body are energetically linked to the feet, as is taught in reflexology, so it's helpful to end a Reiki session by treating the feet. This helps to close the treatment by grounding and centering the client.

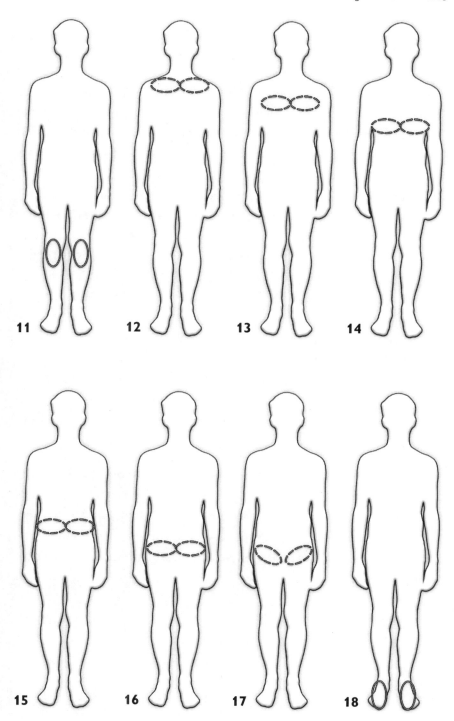

Optional Positions

19. Place one hand at the brow and the other one over the back of the head. Doing so envelops the brain with Reiki energy; it helps calm an overactive mind and treats headache, insomnia, and congestion.

20. The placement of one hand on the brow and one hand at the heart helps instill harmony between one's mental and emotional energies. This combination helps the practitioner instill a sense of heart-mind unity (*kokoro*) in the client.

21. Place one hand at the heart and one over the solar plexus. The lungs, heart, and thymus benefit, as do the stomach and diaphragm. This is one of the most productive measures for treating anxiety, stress, and panic.

22. With your client facing downward (or seated upright), place one hand at their crown and one hand over the base of their spine. This is effective for a quick tune-up, and it leaves the client feeling refreshed, alert, and grounded.

23. As an alternative to hand positions 6 and 7 above, you can treat the left and right sides of the abdomen separately as pictured here. This may be more comfortable for those practitioners whose reach is shorter, making them unable to reach both sides of the body easily from one position. A similar series of hand positions can be used for the back of the client's body.

In the next chapter we will discuss additional, newer Reiki exercises that have evolved over time as Reiki spread through the world. Some of these work with the chakras, and some help treat the *tanden.* Having a variety of exercises at your disposal makes you more marketable as a practitioner, and all of these exercises are useful additions to a fundamental practice.

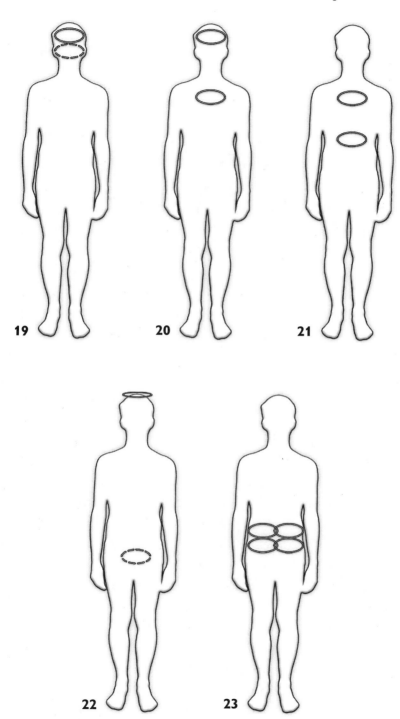

19   20   21

22   23

12

ADDITIONAL REIKI TECHNIQUES

WITH AS MUCH EMPHASIS AS I've placed on tradition, I would be doing a disservice to new Reiki practitioners if I didn't honor the innovation and evolution that the system of Usui Reiki Ryōhō has undergone through transmigration and globalization. Some of the exercises presented in earlier chapters are more recent additions to the system of Reiki Ryōhō that align with the core principles and elements of the system as handed down by Usui.

In this chapter we will explore additional tools and methods for treatment that have been added to the system since the passing of Hawayo Takata in 1980. None of these methods is offered under the pretense of being part of the "original" Reiki teachings. *Dento Reiki* as it is taught in Japan has evolved very slowly and therefore has not incorporated very many new methods. The techniques detailed below largely stem from Western practices; they are helpful ways to augment one's Reiki practice.

In the case that one of the techniques is inspired by or borrowed from a particular lineage, its origins will be noted. However, some of these methods have more diffuse roots, or else they have been adapted or were innovated through my personal practice. Feel free to grow with Reiki by adapting it to suit your own needs and path. When you do so, however, be sure to pass on the whole of the Reiki system, either in a teacher-student relationship or as practitioner to client, and carefully note which aspects fall outside the bounds of Reiki as it was traditionally practiced.

❖ Aura Sweeping

The process of sweeping the human energy field with Reiki is described in brief in chapter 9. It is a gentle means of clearing old patterns or stagnant masses of energy from the aura. Aura-clearing techniques such as this are taught in many styles of Reiki today. Use this method at the end of a treatment of any length of time in order to further propagate Reiki's balancing effects.

1. Connect to Reiki, such as by performing *gasshō meiso*.
2. Once Reiki is flowing, hold your hands over your client, who may be seated, standing, or lying down. Hold your hands about one foot away from your client, and sweep two or three times over the midline of his or her body. Visualize Reiki permeating the aura around your client.
3. Repeat step 2 along the left and right sides of the body. If it is accessible, also sweep through the aura behind your client.
4. Gently beam Reiki to the entire sheath of spiritual energy surrounding your client.
5. Clear your own energy field either with *kenyoku hō* or the Reiki Shower (see chapter 8 for instructions).

❖ Chakra Tune-Up with Reiki

Although people who consider themselves part of the New Age movement may be familiar with the chakras, and practitioners of various spiritual lineages worldwide may be as well, the original Reiki teachings do not make use of the chakras. Since chakras themselves are such an effective means for understanding the subtle energy of human beings, they can be harnessed for a quick and powerful Reiki treatment. (More information on the chakras can be found in appendix A.)

Numerous quick methods of treatment have arisen based upon the chakra system. In my practice, I have found that beginning from the crown and working downward is very grounding, centering, and enlivening. Moving in the other direction, from the base chakra to the crown, is expansive, relaxing, and uplifting for the consciousness. The technique is performed with both client and practitioner standing, but it can be adapted to treat only the front or back of the client if he or she is lying on a massage table.

Note that the hands do not make physical contact with the client during this technique, and the entire process can take less than ten minutes for a full treatment. The downward-moving version of the technique is described below, but the chakras can just as easily be treated in reverse order.

1. Begin in *gasshō* and use your Reiki trigger to initiate the flow of energy.
2. Standing to the side of the recipient, place both hands approximately six inches above the crown chakra. Send Reiki to the crown center for one to two minutes.
3. Place one hand six inches away from the forehead and the other six inches from the back of the skull. Infuse the third-eye chakra with Reiki for one to two minutes.
4. Move to the front and back of the neck in order to treat the throat chakra for one to two minutes.
5. Repeat at the front and back of the heart chakra, located in the middle of the sternum; fill with Reiki for one to two minutes.
6. Treat the solar plexus next, with one hand below the rib cage and the other opposite on the back of the body. Give Reiki for one to two minutes.
7. Treat the sacral chakra, located just below the belly button; the other hand will be opposite at the small of the back.
8. Maintaining a distance of approximately six inches from the body of your client, treat the root chakra with one hand over the groin and the other over the base of the spine.
9. Finish by sweeping through the aura on each side of the recipient.

❂ Treating the Three *Tanden*

Another quick treatment method that is predicated upon a Japanese perspective is treatment of the three *tanden*. The *tanden* are three fields or centers of energy in the body that happen to correlate to the positions of the third-eye, heart, and sacral chakras (although they may not actually be analogous to these energy centers). (Diagrams for all three are located in appendix A.) They may be treated with the client standing, seated, or reclined.

Treating the *tanden* centers is centering, empowering, and revitalizing. The treatment begins at the upper *tanden* and ends at the lower *tanden* because this mimics the natural flow of energy in the body. It also helps restore balance among our spiritual and earthly aspects when the heart is treated, and it finishes by charging up the body's natural battery in the lower *tanden*.

1. Begin in *gasshō* and connect to the flow of Reiki.
2. Place one hand on the brow and treat the upper *tanden* for approximately five minutes.
3. Place both hands on or near the heart in order to treat the middle *tanden* for five minutes.
4. Place one hand on the *hara,* or lower *tanden,* to energize it with Reiki for five minutes.

❂ Meridian Tune-Ups with the Fingers

Usui is likely to have studied the system of meridians used in Chinese medicine, as it was insinuated on the inscription to his memorial stone that he became proficient in such techniques. Although he did not pass this information on in his system of Usui Reiki Ryōhō, an understanding of how the meridians work may have been fundamental to his personal practices, which eventually led to his awakening and achievement of *anshin ritsumei.*

The meridians themselves travel along various points on the body in very specific configurations. Each of the fingers is linked to specific meridians, with points or therapy windows available on each one. These energy pathways can be harnessed for a short treatment. The fingers have many different esoteric correspondences, so treating each of them can balance the elemental constitution, influence the internal organs (as in reflexology), and even balance the chakras.

I first found a similar method, which aims at treating the seven chakras via the fingers, palms, and wrists, in the book *Reiki: The True Story* by Don Beckett.[1] I have simplified the overall process below. Your client may be sitting, standing, or reclining, with palms facing downward.

1. Start by holding your client's thumbs, one in each hand. Allow Reiki to flow for up to five minutes.

2. Move to the index fingers, and treat for the same amount of time.

3. Repeat with the middle fingers.

4. Repeat with the ring fingers.

5. Repeat with the little fingers. This finger opens to two different meridians, one of which is the heart; it may be treated a little longer than the other fingers.

6. Have your client flip his or her hands over so that the palms face upward. Treat both hands in their entirety for up to five minutes.

❖ Reiki Manifestation

In addition to using Reiki to treat people and animals, Reiki is often harnessed to support a variety of circumstances and objects. In the metaphysical community, practitioners send Reiki to their prayers, intentions, vehicles, situations, and lost items. If Reiki is "God power," as Hawayo Takata defined it, then certainly there should be no limit on what it can accomplish. In spite of this, however, there is no historical evidence that Reiki was taught this way before the death of Takata-sensei. No traditional Japanese lineages direct Reiki in this manner, although many styles of Reiki influenced by the New Age movement do.

The mechanics of this technique are very simple, and they are inspired by Mrs. Takata herself. Although she did not teach outright a method of sending Reiki to an intention or situation, she often demonstrated it and talked about it openly.[2] Although a more effective method can be used once the symbols have been introduced in the second degree, or *okuden,* class, level one practitioners can still make use of Reiki for manifestation. Here's how:

1. Begin by visualizing the goal or outcome you would like to manifest. Picture only the end result, leaving the details of *how* it happens up to Reiki.

2. Write down your goal in the form of an affirmation on a piece of paper or index card. Phrase it as a positive statement in the present tense.

3. Hold the card between your hands and practice *gasshō meiso.* While meditating, call upon the higher power(s), however you identify with the

Divine. Ask for divine intervention and the support of Reiki in manifesting your goal.

4. Recite your affirmation, aloud or silently, at least three times while giving the card Reiki between your hands.

5. Express your gratitude (*kanshashite!*) and know that Reiki will support you so long as the outcome is in your best interest.

6. Carry your affirmation or place it in a special place, like a personal altar or shrine, and empower it with Reiki daily.

❂ Charging Crystals with Reiki

Usui-sensei is said to have charged clear quartz crystals with Reiki by giving the crystals *reiju* and giving those stones to clients who lived far away. The crystals themselves held the Reiki energy and could be placed directly on the body for healing when a Reiki practitioner was not available. Today, this practice has been adapted so that practitioners of all levels can empower quartz and other minerals with the healing force of Reiki.

Begin with an already cleansed crystal; varieties of quartz tend to work best, although you can select another stone that suits your situation. Reiki-charged crystals will need to be re-empowered in time, because the following method is not permanent like initiations are. After charging it, place your crystal in a purse or pocket to carry with you, leave it in a room that could benefit from uplifting energy, gift it to someone in need of healing, or sit it atop your affirmation card to enhance your Reiki manifestation.

1. Connect to Reiki in a manner that is meaningful for you.

2. Hold your crystal between your palms in *gasshō* and visualize Reiki bathing the stone in radiant light. As you inhale, picture Reiki flowing from the universe into your crown and down to your *hara*. As you exhale, allow Reiki to rise from the *hara* and travel down your arms and hands and into the stone.

3. Recite the *gokai* three times so that the *kotodama* of these words infuses the crystal with the core ideals of the Reiki system.

4. When you are finished, thank the crystal (and Reiki) for co-creating with you in this process.

5. Recharge the stone at least once a week, or more often if you feel as though the energy has dissipated.

✪ Opening and Closing Spiral

The Opening and Closing Spirals are simple tools that may be incorporated into your standard treatment as a means of enhancing the effects of Reiki. Originating in the work of the late author and medical doctor W. Brugh Joy, the meditation was adapted to a Reiki treatment method by John Harvey Gray, one of Hawayo Takata's twenty-two teachers. He first describes the technique in his book *Hand to Hand*. It has grown in popularity, especially in the Reiki communities of New England.

John writes that using the Opening Spiral "jump-starts the energy-delivery cycle and helps the client utilize more Reiki for healing purposes."[3] It is usually employed after scanning or after the practitioner has otherwise checked the health of the energy field (such as in *byōsen reikan hō*) and prior to *chiryō,* or hands-on healing.

The Closing Spiral is the same technique applied in reverse. The closing procedure serves as a means of sealing the session, and it "is enormously helpful in supporting clients to hold the energy so the healing process will continue after the session is over."[4] Most practitioners who use the Closing Spiral follow it with an aura-clearing procedure, such as Aura Sweeping described above. I have simplified both the Opening and Closing Spirals to include only the seven major chakras, the feet, and the transpersonal point above the crown center. Please refer to *Hand to Hand* or a teacher in the Takata-Gray lineage for the expanded version of this technique.

Opening Spiral Instructions

1. Begin with your hand just above the client's heart chakra. Give Reiki in this position for up to fifteen seconds, just enough to stimulate the energy center.
2. Moving in a clockwise motion, continue to treat each chakra for up to fifteen seconds in the following order: heart, solar plexus, throat, sacral, third-eye, root, and crown chakras, below the feet (earth star chakra), and transpersonal point above the crown (soul star chakra). Refer to the

diagram in appendix A (page 287) for the location of the seven major chakras; the remaining two chakras lie approximately one foot below the feet (earth star chakra) and one foot above the head (soul star chakra).

Closing Spiral Instructions

1. Begin with your hand at the transpersonal point above the crown. Give Reiki at this point for up to fifteen seconds.
2. Moving counterclockwise, continue from the transpersonal point to the other energy centers in the reverse order of the Opening Spiral: below the feet (earth star chakra), and then the crown, root, third-eye, sacral, throat, solar plexus, and heart chakras.

❂ Expanding Your Light

In traditional Reiki Ryōhō, students are taught several different meditative exercises meant to increase their capacity to channel Reiki. Usui devised these methods in order to help laypeople reach *anshin ritsumei* as he could, and to supercharge students' sensitivity to *byōsen*. The actual techniques vary from one lineage to another. Takata-sensei referred to these practices, collectively called *hatsurei hō* (which means "method for increasing *rei* or spirit"), in a journal entry dated December 10, 1935.[5]

I usually teach the formal method of *hatsurei hō* in the *okuden* class. However, as a means of giving new practitioners a viable tool to improve their Reiki practice, the following meditation is presented. It resembles a technique called Light Breathing that's used in Gendai Reiki Hō and in shamanic Reiki. A simple meditation, it can be practiced for as little as five minutes or for as long as the practitioner likes.

With regular practice, Light Breathing or any other adaptation of *hatsurei hō* will refine your entire being as a vessel for Reiki. It is naturally a purifying practice, and it will help stubborn patterns of disharmony dissipate over time. It is a wonderful tool to prepare you for the second degree initiation.

1. Hold your hands in *gasshō* and connect to the flow of Reiki. You may use the Chalice Meditation or Reiki Shower to increase the flow of Reiki in your energy field.

2. Holding your hands in *gasshō,* imagine that every breath carries bright white light, in addition to oxygen, into your lungs.

3. Allow the light to expand outward from your chest as you exhale. Imagine that disharmony, resistance to the light, and stagnant areas are transformed by the white light of Reiki.

4. Continue this visualization until you are ready to end your meditation.

This wraps up part 1 of the book. In part 2 we will explore *okuden,* or second degree Reiki, as well as enter into a discussion of the very important Reiki symbols. We will then go on to explore other Reiki techniques and various other components of a successful Reiki practice.

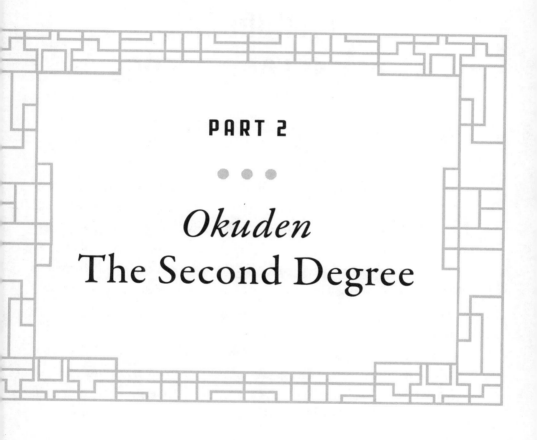

PART 2

· · ·

Okuden
The Second Degree

13

INTRODUCING THE SECOND DEGREE

THE SECOND DEGREE of Usui Reiki Ryōhō imparts new tools to the practitioner. It is first and foremost a step toward deepening our relationship with Reiki itself. Most practitioners of Reiki eventually move to the second degree because of the enhanced power, expanded techniques, and broader reach that this training provides for clients. Its benefits reach far beyond the application of physical healing and self-healing. It equips practitioners with a series of effective tools for virtually every condition or situation.

In the original Reiki teachings, the second degree is called *okuden.* Originally written as 奥傳, *okuden* means "the inner teachings" of Reiki Ryōhō. In *shoden,* new practitioners receive initiations or attunements to grant them the initial experience of Reiki within themselves, thus conferring the ability to harness Reiki energy for healing. In the second level of the Usui System of Natural Healing, practitioners are again initiated, and they are taught the sacred symbols for enhancing treatments.

Shoden can be thought of as opening the doors to Reiki practice; hence its name translates as "entrance teachings." *Okuden,* however, is stepping inside the room and taking advantage of all the possibilities therein. In viewing the progressive degrees of Reiki in this manner, we see that they build upon one another in a meaningful way that facili-

216

tates personal development and growth on behalf of the practitioners.

The second degree refines the quality of the Reiki that's available to channel. Level two practitioners undergo further *reiju,* or initiations, in order to purify and strengthen their capacities as conduits for Reiki. The traditional forms of Reiki in Japan use a single *reiju* ritual; it's the same for each level. Here in the West, branches of Reiki derived from Takata-sensei generally utilize a different ceremony for each degree; thus the symbols of the second degree are empowered through the ritual itself.

LEARNING THE SECOND DEGREE

Taking the training for *okuden* should happen at a pace with which you feel comfortable. In Usui's time only those candidates who were proficient at sensing *byōsen* and could successfully perform *reiji hō* were permitted to enroll in the next seminar. This might mean waiting years between the two levels. Ideally, whenever you receive your initiation into the second degree, you should be committed to the practice and precepts of the Reiki tradition.

As mentioned earlier in this book, one of the innovations that Hayashi Chūjirō brought to Reiki Ryōhō was teaching *shoden* and *okuden* together. Doing so made it possible for students to take the entire training at once, a practice especially beneficial when travel was necessary in order to become a Reiki practitioner. Nowadays, this convention is very popular; many Reiki teachers offer weekend seminars or courses of a week's duration that combine the first and second degrees into one extended seminar.

Hawayo Takata, on the other hand, insisted that the majority of her students wait before taking the second degree. She preferred for students to gain as much practice as possible before advancing so that the core competencies of the first degree were fully integrated into her students' experiences. There is no wrong time to learn, so long as students are diligent in using Reiki, adhere to the Five Principles, and are willing to grow.

The training itself in *okuden* is simpler in many ways than the training in *shoden* because students are already familiar with Reiki. Discussing history, energy basics, and the fundamental practices is unnecessary because they were covered in the previous level. Instead, the second degree mostly focuses on the symbols and how to apply them.

CORE ELEMENTS OF THE SECOND DEGREE

The six elements of Reiki discussed in chapter 1 are equally as relevant to the second degree. The only part of this list untouched in the *shoden* class is the use of the symbols and mantras themselves. The initiation, *gokai,* and use of Reiki treatments are all expanded through the second degree, as is personal development. Thus, it might be desirable to include a basic review of these elements to serve as a refresher before moving into new territory for students.

The Reiki symbols themselves fall into categories of *shirushi,* or primal symbols, and *jumon,* or formulas of words that will be discussed in greater detail in the coming chapters. The symbols become the platform for the new practices introduced in the second degree, including mental-emotional healing and distance treatments.

In addition to learning the symbols, in *okuden* we learn how to treat our own psyche and that of others. While the tools offered in the first degree are predominantly focused on self-healing and healing at the physical level, the symbols broaden the scope of Reiki's efficacy. We can learn to treat conditions beginning in our hearts and minds and those of our clients through the use of the *okuden* techniques. Learning to heal across any distance is also a major aspect of an *okuden* class. One of the symbols facilitates this process; it fosters the ability of Reiki practitioners to connect more deeply to the recipients of Reiki despite separation by physical distance, time, or any other limitation.

Other tools include enhancing the net effect of Reiki, as the symbols and meditations in *okuden* increase the overall efficacy of treatments. *Okuden* endows practitioners with an effective means of focusing the infinite blessings of Reiki onto a specific target, thus supporting them in becoming more effective at treating *byōsen.* The second degree also allows practitioners to send Reiki to more esoteric targets, such as goals, groups of people, situations, and/or specific places.

Choosing to participate in the *okuden* class helps you grow with Reiki. It is a helpful step if you're interested in practicing Reiki professionally or if you want to bring your healing into new frontiers. The symbols and techniques that practitioners learn in *okuden* are catalysts for deeper and more profound healing, and they propel you further along the Reiki path.

RAISING YOUR CONSCIOUSNESS

One of the common themes that arises in *okuden* training is the emphasis on personal development. The symbols themselves are transcendental tools for attaining greater mastery over the self and a deeper, more surrendered connection to the source of Reiki. By cultivating the skills and concepts embodied in the second degree, we approach the unknowable; this is the meaning of the inner teachings of *okuden*.

In Reiki Ryōhō, the ultimate goal is realization of *anshin ritsumei*, a state of indescribable peace in which our life purpose can be accomplished. Apart from the life path that we make in the material world, which is unique to each person, we all share the same spiritual purpose. Our one goal for spiritual attainment is union with Source. This is described in different religions and spiritual paths in many ways, and in Japan it's often associated as becoming one with kami, the essence of the Divine.

Usui Reiki Ryōhō is one means of accomplishing the goal of connecting to and becoming inseparable from Source. The symbols themselves repeatedly point to the idea that Reiki energy is a direct effect of the highest order of Creation—the consciousness of the Divine—acting on the physical plane. Reiki is a tool that works as an intermediary between the worlds of Kami Consciousness (or Buddha Consciousness or Christ Consciousness) and the mind of humankind. The symbols work as specific tools for bringing us into alignment with the higher realms to heal at the most profound levels available.

Now let's take a closer look at the use of symbols in Reiki practice.

14

THE REIKI SYMBOLS

THREE SACRED SYMBOLS are incorporated into Reiki Ryōhō at the *okuden* level.* Each has a specific function, which has precise effects when used during a treatment. Due to the information age in which we live, the symbols can be found virtually anywhere one looks, from websites to CDs, in books and on jewelry—they even appear as tattoos! Out of respect for tradition, I've decided to maintain the convention of not revealing the symbols themselves in this text, although their form, origin, and names (or mantras) will be described alongside their applications.

Symbols in general evoke a reaction on our primal, subconscious levels. They speak to the inner depths of the mind and soul and help to invite a particular feeling or energy. The symbols used in Reiki have their origins in Japanese culture, and they were added to facilitate specific aspects of healing and spiritual growth. Before we delve into what they are, let's first describe some terms that are used to discuss them.

In Western branches of Reiki, there isn't much separation between the different categories of Reiki symbols. However, in Japan, the nature

---

*The following chapters will make frequent comparisons between the symbols of Western and Japanese styles of Reiki Ryōhō. However, please note that the symbols used in my classes, and therefore described at length in this text, are *only* those of the Western lineages. Discussions of the symbols' original forms and uses are provided to gain an accurate historical context and to better understand the mechanisms behind the functions of each of them. (If you would like training in the original uses of the symbols, please enroll in a Jikiden Reiki seminar near you for *shoden* and *okuden*.)

of the symbols is more apparent, especially in the case of the distance healing symbol, which is comprised of kanji. The first two symbols, referred to as the power symbol (or focus symbol) and the mental-emotional healing symbol (or the harmony symbol), are considered *shirushi*. The word *shirushi*, or 印, simply means "sign," "mark," or "symbol" in Japanese. In Usui Reiki Ryōhō it conveys the meaning of being a primordial energy all its own. The power of *shirushi* lies in simply drawing it, and for this reason Japanese styles of Reiki do not use an accompanying mantra with these two symbols.

The third symbol, which is used in long-distance healing, is considered to be a *jumon*. This word, written 呪文 in kanji, is usually rendered in English as "spell," "incantation," or "magic formula." *Jumon* refers to the formulaic composition of characters, typically kanji, constructed for a specific spiritual or ritual purpose. The power of a *jumon* in the system of Reiki lies in the spoken word; the symbols themselves are merely everyday characters or kanji. They produce an effect because of the strong *kotodama* that animates them. Although some Western writers use the word *jumon* to refer to the accompanying mantra or recitation of the symbols' names as is practiced in Western lineages of Reiki, the more correct term would be *shingon* or even *kotodama*.

To revisit the idea of *kotodama*, it's important to understand that the Japanese believe that there is a vital power inherent in sounds. *Kotodama* (言靈) is literally the "soul of words" or the "spiritual vibration carried by sounds." All sounds have *kotodama*, but specific words invoke stronger effects when used consciously. This is the purpose behind reciting the *gokai* in Japanese, as well as the reason for speaking a *jumon* aloud. Even in Westernized forms of Reiki, speaking the names of the symbols out loud invokes the *kotodama* in their names.

The word in Japanese for mantra is *shingon*, written 真言. This expression literally means "true words." (*Shingon* also refers to a sect of Buddhism that makes heavy use of esoteric teachings and tools, such as mantras.) In the case of Usui Shiki Ryōhō and other styles influenced by it, the names of the symbols are used as *shingon*. The mantra helps empower and focus one's attention, even though this is not required to "activate" the symbol itself. The original Japanese schools of Reiki do not employ the *shingon* of *shirushi,* at least not at the second degree. One doesn't have to recite the name of a spoon or hammer to make it work. In the same way, the original Japanese schools of Reiki found it unnecessary to recite the names of the symbols themselves.

The development of the mantra recitation with the Reiki symbols was introduced by Hawayo Takata. Since she left virtually no written instructions behind, it is unclear exactly how this practice changed over time. The most likely case is that the addition of the mantras is a simplification of the *kotodama* used in the psychological treatment; this method requires the practitioner to recite a long command, originally in Japanese. Takata-sensei would have needed a way to simplify and standardize the symbol usage for Western audiences. Since the third symbol, really a *jumon,* already required the repetition of the symbol's name, the practice seeped into the use of the other two symbols as well.

THE ORIGINS OF THE REIKI SYMBOLS

As we have learned, in 1922 Reiki's founder Usui Mikao had a revelatory experience on Mount Kurama in which the ability to connect to Reiki was transmitted to him from the universe. When he eventually chose to share his ability with others, the symbols were added in order to facilitate the experience of practicing Reiki. Remember that most of us are not planning to fast until we die atop a holy mountain, so Usui Reiki Ryōhō makes use of tools that enable an ordinary person to aspire to Usui's level of proficiency. These tools include *reiju,* the *gokai,* and the *shirushi* and *jumon.*

The symbols themselves have older roots, such as in Shinto and Buddhism. Usui chose common themes and simplified them for the layperson. Because of this, the symbols were made to be used only within the context of Usui Reiki Ryōhō. To the uninitiated, they would mean very little. It's likely that the symbols were not a part of Usui's original teachings, though they were probably introduced to the system of Reiki soon thereafter, around the time that a formal initiation procedure was developed.

After nearly a century, the symbols have noticeably changed. Because traditions maintain that the symbols are respected and reserved for the initiated only, they are not written down in early texts about Reiki. Even today in some traditional lineages from Japan the symbols are not written down or handed out by teachers. Since students are expected to memorize them, their forms have naturally been modified over generations of practitioners.

The simpler forms often have the greatest amount of variation, especially arising after the proliferation of Reiki when Hawayo Takata passed away. Variances in handwriting can easily be mistaken for the literal form of the symbols themselves in a culture that cannot read Japanese nor has any familiarity with the inspiration behind the symbols. Because of the inordinate number of different versions of each symbol, many Reiki *shihan* and practitioners are moving toward standardization by checking their symbols against historic sources.

SECRET OR SACRED?

In Japan today, the three second degree symbols are kept secret, mostly because they have been adapted to suit the needs of practitioners. Since Usui-sensei simplified other spiritual teachings and made them available in his Reiki Ryōhō, the symbols would not be recognizable to outsiders. This, when combined with the overall nature of the Japanese to maintain the rules of their groups and organizations, is largely why the *shirushi* and *jumon* are kept under wraps in Japan.

When Reiki was brought to the Americas, the symbols were considered a trade secret; they were only to be shared among practitioners. Takata-sensei taught her students that the symbols had no power of their own if the person receiving them had not undergone initiation into Reiki. Take notice of the difference here: Japanese styles teach that the symbols have no *value* to a nonpractitioner who wouldn't understand their use, whereas Takata taught the symbols had no *effect* for the uninitiated.

Hawayo Takata typically did not permit students to take any drawings of the symbols home from her classes. This too contributed to the high degree of variation of the symbols used by successive generations of teachers and students. Since the 1990s, dozens of books have been published that contain the symbols, often in forms unrecognizable to practitioners of *dento Reiki.*

Although there is a convention of secrecy surrounding the symbols, we can shift our focus and consider them sacred. Sacred images, such as icons or statues, are treated with deference and piety. Although Reiki is not a religion, it is deeply spiritual; the symbols, therefore, can be considered holy in their own right. By placing the Reiki symbols in the realm of the sacred, we may embrace a treatment of them that honors their origins, traditions, and powerful effects.

The *jumon* and *shirushi* of the Reiki system are powerful tools. They should not be taken lightly—they command respect and a certain degree of reverence. Generally, one should not place them in public places, wear them as jewelry, or openly draw or pronounce their *shingon* where others will notice.

WORKING WITH THE SYMBOLS

Usui-sensei and those who practice *dento Reiki* have very specific indications for the use of each symbol. They are often applied only in a single manner each time they're used. Viewed through the lens of a Japanese perspective, this is simply the way things are and the way they have been since our esteemed founder created Reiki. The Western mind, however, likes to innovate and sometimes holds onto the tools themselves more than the message underlying their outer forms. Thus, the symbols have been given a multitude of uses as Reiki migrated from culture to culture.

Initially, the simplest way to get to know the symbols is by drawing them again and again. Since they must be memorized in order to be used effectively, practicing them in this way serves two purposes: Drawing the *shirushi* and *jumon* helps establish a clear relationship to them, and it makes it easy to recall them during treatments.

Due to the fact that the symbols are very powerful, they are used sparingly in the original forms of Reiki. Among Western traditions, however, the symbols have been subjected to trial-and-error experimentation to find additional applications for them. One of the most profound ways to use the symbols is to employ them during the practice of meditation. They may be drawn or visualized, or their accompanying mantras may be recited as one enters the meditative state. The symbols themselves will guide the user of them to their true meaning and purpose.

Use the symbols on yourself repeatedly before applying them on your clients or loved ones. Build an intimate relationship with the symbols so that you can anticipate their effects on others. They may be used in a variety of ways, such as to empower crystals, to bless food or gifts, to clear the energy of a room, and/or to offer protection and safety during travel. Of course, they are first and foremost meant to be used for our healing and personal development, so they are best used in meditation and during hands-on treatments.

Whenever the symbols are drawn (enacted), they alter or augment the quality of the Reiki, almost as though the lens through which one sees its effects is being changed. The symbols act as cosmic seeds of force; they are antennas that conduct a specific wavelength or archetype of energy for healing and evolution. Because of this, the symbols are powerful and offer profound healing on all levels.

When drawing a symbol with your hand in the air or over a client you are working on, it's best to hold all of your fingers close together, rather than using a single finger to delineate the symbol. If drawing over a smaller area, use the index and middle fingers together, because, as we have established, the middle finger emits the strongest energy. Symbols can also be drawn with the palm of the hand very discreetly during hands-on healing, without even removing your hands from the client's body. Use whichever method works best for you according to the lineage of Reiki Ryōhō that you practice.

In addition to simply *drawing* the symbols, a multitude of ways to access their benefits have been explored in Western styles of Reiki. You can try any of the following methods and compare the results:

- Visualize the symbols in your mind or on the recipient.
- Chant their names/mantras aloud.
- Recite the names/mantras silently.
- Draw them on the roof of your mouth with your tongue.
- Picture the symbols on the palms of your hands when giving treatment.
- Silently ask for the intervention of the energy of the symbols.

Remember that the symbols themselves are inherently empty; our intention and connection to Reiki comprise the real tools at our disposal. For this reason, the *shirushi* and *jumon* are meant to be used as training wheels; with enough practice we can let them go. Approaching the symbols in this way prepares us to *become* the symbols. We empty ourselves of attachment and expectation in order to integrate the message they point us toward.

Next we will look at the symbols themselves.

15

THE FIRST SYMBOL:
CHOKU REI

OF THE THREE SYMBOLS taught in the practitioner level of Reiki Ryōhō, the *choku rei* is by far the simplest. In Japanese, its name is written with the kanji 直靈. These characters together can be interpreted as "direct transmission of spirit." A popular though incorrect etymology used in Western branches of Reiki translates the expression *choku rei* as "imperial decree," using the characters 勅令, which are pronounced the same way. Although these kanji may form a more common expression in Japanese, the correct name of the first *shirushi* is written with the characters 直靈.

Other meanings for *choku rei* include:

- direct spirit
- true soul
- true energy of the universe
- creators of mankind
- spirits directly begotten by God
- correct spirit
- fixed spirit

The name of this symbol can also be read with alternate pronunciations: *naohi* and *naobi*. They are simply alternate ways to read the same kanji (直靈). The expressions *naohi* and *naobi* are used in Shinto and aikido, pointing to a very ancient origin of this symbol's context. It is important to note that only the *name,* and thus its *kotodama* or mantra, is found in these traditions as *naohi/naobi.* The symbol itself is an original creation of Usui Mikao.

In most forms of Reiki, the *choku rei* is known as the power symbol, for it increases the efficacy of, or powers up, the treatment. Some Eastern branches refer to it as the focus symbol, whereas others only refer to it by its calligraphic origins, which will be discussed below.

ORIGINS

The first Reiki symbol is regarded as a *shirushi* in Japanese lineages. This means that it's a primordial form with its own soul or intelligence. Power from the *shirushi* is evoked when their outer forms are drawn or merely visualized. Therefore, they don't require the spoken word or *kotodama* to generate their effects. Usui simplified complex teachings and symbols in his system of Usui Reiki Ryōhō. Considering this, the use of *choku rei* as a mantra embodying the *kotodama* of this symbol is likely to have started in the West, rather than in Japan.[1]

The *choku rei,* or power symbol, combines the ancient idea of the *naohi* with the shape of a beautiful spiral figure. Spiraling forms are common throughout the world. They often convey a message of movement, energy, transformation, and change, as well as the cyclical nature of time. The *choku rei* clearly signifies energy and movement, even though it's Usui's original work. Spirals are frequent motifs in early shamanic cultures, including Shinto.

The actual shape of the power symbol is derived from Japanese calligraphy and rooted in Shinto beliefs. Although the spiral itself is a universal symbol, the external form of this *shirushi* is actually derived from a kanji. It is taken from the radical for rain, called *ame,* and is written 雨 in normal script. The *ame* radical is found in other kanji, including the words for "spirit" (*rei* 靈), "snow" (*yuki* 雪), "cloud" (*kumo* 雲), "thunder" (*kaminari* 雷), and "fog" (*kiri* 霧). Each of these words has a heavenly or

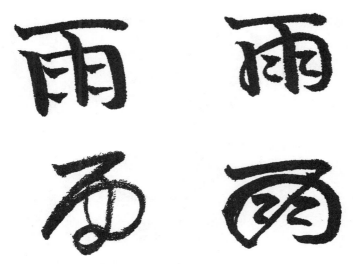

Here, *ame,* the character meaning "rain," is written in several styles.
Moving clockwise from the top left, this character becomes
more cursive and begins to spiral like the *choku rei.*
Calligraphy by author

immaterial connotation; they come from the celestial planes. In a similar fashion, the first *shirushi* also "signifies the highest place, that which humans cannot reach which is the source of Reiki."[2]

The spiral form of the *choku rei* shares its roots with the artistic motif of the "auspicious cloud." Called *xiang yun* in Chinese and *zui un* in Japanese (瑞雲), this common visual motif is a spiraling cloud shape. It is used to represent good fortune, blessings, and the heavenly forces at work. Like the meaning of the *ame* radical in the kanji for *rei* (see chapter 1), the underlying symbolism of the *zui un* is of the heavenly blessings raining down.* Given that the characters for both *cloud* and *rain* appear to be very similar when written in cursive script, either is a possible source of the outer shape of the *choku rei.*

---

*It's an interesting correlation to note that the auspicious cloud motif frequently appears in Chinese iconography as part of the *ruyi* scepter, which is held to represent authority. It may lend a vague connection to the translation of *choku rei* as "imperial decree," for *ruyi* means "as one wishes"—whatever one commands will be carried out. The cloud motif is used on the scepter to support the idea that the blessings of the heavens will enact one's desires.

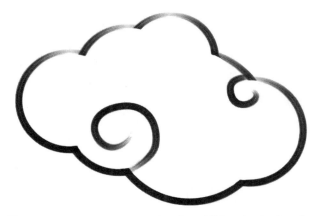

The *zui un,* or auspicious cloud, exhibits a spiraling form like that of the *choku rei.*

The mantra or name of *choku rei* is not used in Japanese Reiki except in rare circumstances, where it is pronounced *naohi* or *naobi.* In fact, Reiki researcher and *shihan* Nishina Masaki notes the differences between the first *shirushi* of Jikiden and Western Reiki, saying, "A similar form is used in Japanese Reiki but for different purposes and on different occasions. Therefore, using [*choku* rei] like this is something Takata developed incorrectly in terms of Japanese Reiki. The mantra connected to [this symbol] in Western Reiki, *choku rei,* is actually an incorrect reading of the original kanji characters 直靈. These characters can be read correctly if one has knowledge of Shinto. It is very puzzling that Takata taught it incorrectly."[3]

The use of *naohi* or 直靈 is also found in aikido, Oomoto, and Shinto practices in Japan. In these contexts, *naohi/naobi* describes the action in which the kami breathed life into Earth during the act of Creation. Human beings developed from this life force or soul (靈) and thus are directly connected to the kami or divine being(s). In Japan it is generally believed that this soul is implanted into developing babies while they are in utero, placed within the upper *tanden* by the kami themselves. Thus, within humanity "works the life-giving power (*choku rei*), that is sent directly from the gods through the crown into the center of human beings."[4]

To the Japanese, the idea of the human soul or spirit is described as *ichirei shikon* (一靈四魂). *Ichirei* means "one soul," and *shikon* translates as "four spirits."* The four component spirits or souls are called the *kushitama* (奇魂, "wondrous soul"), *aratama* (荒魂, "rough soul"), *nigitama* (和魂, "harmonious soul"), and *sakitama* (幸魂, "happy soul"). Collectively, these four essential qualities comprise the *naohi/naobi* (直靈) or *reikon* (靈魂).

The four souls of the human being, as described in Shintoism, are nourished by the inner god force, or *choku rei/naohi.*[5] Remember from chapter 1 that there are many varieties of ki, and that the highest order is called *shinki* (神氣), or the *ki of the kami* (gods/divine beings). However, *shinki* is too rarefied to act directly on the material plane, so Reiki is the next highest order of ki, which enacts the mission of the kami in our world. The *choku rei* symbol gives us a direct transmission of the Divine or heavenly energy, here visualized as *ame* or spiritual rain, so that we can focus this energy at the material level for healing. In using the *shirushi choku rei*, we are tapping into the same nourishing power of the soul, or *naohi*, itself.

The external form of the *choku rei* symbol has evolved over the generations of Reiki practitioners since Usui. The direction of the spiral and its number of turns have been altered many times. Even the symbol as Takata-sensei taught it was slightly different from those used in *dento Reiki* and changed over the years that she taught.

UNDERSTANDING THE *CHOKU REI*: POWER SYMBOL OR FOCUS SYMBOL?

Takata's style of Reiki Ryōhō and those branches descended from it use the first symbol as means of amplifying the energy used during treatment, thereby cutting treatment time in half. For this reason, it

---

*Because of the esoteric and often vague nature of the Japanese language, the terms *rei* (靈) and *kon* (魂) are often substituted for one another, and their meanings overlap. Thus, *ichirei shikon* can mean both "one soul, four spirits" *and* "one spirit, four souls." To complicate matters further, both 魂 and 靈 can be read as *tama,* making it very easy to confuse the two characters and their precise meanings.

is simply called the power symbol by most practitioners on those occasions when speaking its proper name/mantra is not ideal. Folk etymologies in these branches of Reiki sometimes translate *choku rei* as "put the power here," which closely resembles the action of this symbol from the perspective of *dento Reiki.*

If we look at Takata-sensei's correspondence with her Reiki student American heiress Doris Duke, we see that Takata provides a short lesson on this symbol in a letter dated December 1978. In it, Takata states that the *choku rei* "means to command all Reiki scattered in the universe to gather immediately on the area you treat."[6] Although Takata goes on to say that this symbol "increases your power into 100 horsepower, so the treatment results are faster," we can see that she isn't describing a mechanism that merely adds power. Instead, the *choku rei* condenses or focuses energy to a specific point.[7]

In some schools of Japanese Reiki and in hybrids of Eastern and Western approaches, the first symbol is called the "focus symbol." Rather than increasing the flow of Reiki through the practitioner, the *choku rei* "pinpoints the shape, matter, and substance, and condenses and sends strong energy to it."[8] In other words, it directs (直) the spiritual energy (靈) into a concise point of focus to harness it at the material level of existence at which we dwell. Japanese forms of Reiki typically reserve this *shirushi* primarily for applications of physical healing.

The spiral contained in the form of the *choku rei* symbol directs the heavenly blessings (or *ame*) during the treatment. The horizontal line at the top of the figure represents the heavenly or spiritual energy, which descends upon us with the vertical stroke. Finally, the inward-moving spiral moves the flow of the heavenly Reiki from a diffuse rain to a condensed point. The effect of drawing this symbol creates a vortex, or spiral of energy, that reaches down from the highest realms to the point at which it is drawn.

Whether you subscribe to the belief that this *shirushi* is a power increase or a focus point, the end result is the same. In aikido, the *naobi* is known to have a similar effect: "when Naobi [直靈], direct spirit, comes into activity, various high frequency light wave vibrations are emanated."⁹ The increase in power described by Western lineages of Reiki is really the effect of the heavenly resources of Reiki energy converging where the *choku rei* is drawn.

USING *CHOKU REI*

In treatments, the first *shirushi* increases the flow of Reiki. In hands-on treatments, this means that you can become a conduit for a greater amount of Reiki on behalf of your clients. When the symbol is drawn, it's as if the universe is conspiring to pour healing energy into the point at which it is drawn. It is helpful to draw this symbol at the beginning of a session; it will improve the efficacy of the entire treatment.

You can also draw the *choku rei* on your hands, body, and/or chakras as a means of increasing the amount of Reiki flowing through you during treatment. The overall effect of the *choku rei* is purifying and grounding, which enables you as a practitioner to be a more effective vessel through which Reiki can flow. Drawing it in your own energy field can increase the magnitude of your aura, making it more resistant to outside influences. For this reason, some branches of Reiki use it to provide protection.

Japanese forms of practice have a different *shirushi* in place of *choku rei*. It is morphologically similar although the indications are distinct. Jikiden Reiki preserves this *shirushi* as Hayashi-sensei taught it (which is presumably the same way that Usui did, too), and its sole use is for targeting *byōsen*. Nishina explains the difference between the *choku rei* and the Japanese *shirushi*, telling us that since *byōsen* "was not taught in the Western system of Reiki, the shirushi for [*byōsen*] was not taught either. It is important not to make the mistake of thinking this *shirushi* is [*choku rei*], which came from an entirely different *shirushi*."*¹⁰

---

*This passage from Nishina's work, as well as the writings of Jikiden founder Yamaguchi Tadao and bestselling Reiki author Frank Arjava Petter, seem to indicate that the *choku rei* is in fact a separate *shirushi* altogether. At the time of writing, I am currently unsure whether it has a counterpart in *dento Reiki* (as I suspect), or if it evolved independently via Takata's adaptations to the system of Reiki Ryōhō.

Whenever resistance or disharmony is encountered, which is experienced as different levels of *byōsen,* the focus symbol may be drawn to create an uprising of energy to break up the source of disharmony. The symbol itself can be drawn almost imperceptibly without lifting the hand(s) so that the client is unaware that a symbol is being drawn. Using the *choku rei* in this manner therefore cuts treatment time in half, just as Takata-sensei taught her students. After speaking with many other practitioners of Western Reiki, including those who have knowledge of the techniques used in Jikiden Reiki, I was surprised at the number of people who intuitively use *choku rei* in this manner.

In general, the *choku rei* can be employed anytime you need to concentrate or increase the flow of Reiki to a specific location. It can be used for *heso chiryō, tanden chiryō,* or any hands-on healing method, especially when you encounter *byōsen.*

Additional Uses

Western Reiki has always had a flair for innovation, and it is through the trial-and-error approach that many practitioners and teachers have found additional applications of the Reiki symbols. Because of the relative ease and simplicity of drawing the *choku rei,* it is the symbol most frequently applied outside of traditional methods.

Try using the power symbol to:

- bless food, beverages, or gifts
- clear and cleanse rooms of disharmony by drawing on the walls, ceiling, and floor
- prepare yourself for giving or receiving a Reiki treatment
- promote grounding by drawing the symbol on the soles of the feet
- treat faulty appliances, electronics, and other household objects
- seal and anchor the positive effects after a treatment by drawing over a person's heart or *hara*
- empower or increase the energy of other Reiki symbols

❖ Strengthening Your Lightbody

The following technique uses the *choku rei* as a tool to increase one's personal power. When it is drawn in the aura and over the chakras, one's inner conduit for Reiki is supercharged. The *choku rei* will help cleanse and align the body's energy centers as well, helping to improve overall well-being, reduce negative influences from one's surroundings, and increase sensitivity to the needs of clients during treatment. It helps strengthen the energy field or lightbody all around. If one is unable to practice this method in privacy, the name or mantra may be recited in the mind.

1. Begin with your hands in *gasshō,* and await the flow of Reiki.
2. Draw the symbol on each of your hands, recite its mantra three times, and tap your hands together with three gentle claps.
3. Draw a large *choku rei* in front of you. Make it big enough to reach from your head to your hips. Motion with your hands to draw it toward you as you recite its mantra three times.
4. Beginning with the root chakra, draw a small *choku rei* and move it into the chakra. Recite its name once as you do so.
5. Repeat step 4 for the remaining chakras.

❖ Creating Sacred Space

As an alternative or addition to reciting the *gokai* for clearing the energy of a space, the *choku rei* can be drawn on the walls to fill a room with the heavenly blessings of Reiki. Once that is done, the other symbols can be drawn in the center of the room as a means of broadcasting their healing presence into each part of one's sacred space.

1. Begin in *gasshō.* Prepare yourself by performing the technique Expanding Your Light.
2. Draw the *choku rei* in the air over each wall and recite its mantra three times for each time it is drawn.
3. Stand in the center of the room and raise your hands upward; draw the symbol, and picture it being drawn on the ceiling. Recite the mantra three times.
4. Repeat the same actions for the floor.

5. Draw the *choku rei* symbol in the air in the center of the room and recite its mantra. Repeat with the *sei heki* (second symbol) and *hon sha ze shō nen* (third symbol).

❖ Sealing the Treatment

When I first learned Reiki, my teacher offered a powerful tool for ending a hands-on treatment by sealing the positive changes with the *choku rei.* This is a simple way to anchor the progress that Reiki has made, and it prevents the client from backsliding once he or she resumes normal activities. Western in origin, sealing your treatments helps the positive change root itself more deeply for lasting benefits.

1. When finished with your normal treatment procedures, sweep through the aura and place the hands six to ten inches over the *tanden* or solar plexus.
2. Beam Reiki to the center of the client's body, visualizing it spreading throughout the energy field.
3. Draw the *choku rei* and silently recite its mantra three times.
4. Mentally or aloud affirm that the healing process is sealed in divine love, using whatever words are the most meaningful to you.

The next chapter will detail the second symbol, *sei heki.*

16

THE SECOND SYMBOL: *SEI HEKI*

THE SECOND *OKUDEN* SYMBOL is used for psychological healing; it is called *sei heki* in Western lineages of Reiki. *Sei heki* is written as 性 癖 in Japanese, which means "bad habit" or "vice" in modern Japanese. Traditionally, Western lineages of Reiki have considered the *sei heki* to be the mental/emotional healing symbol, which is derived from its earliest use in Japan.

Sei or 性 is a combination of the radicals for "heart" (*kokoro*), which is simplified in this word, and the root for "birth." It's often translated as "the inherent nature of something," such as a person's sex or gender. The roots of this word may be said to represent "the heart of one's nature from birth"; these are the fundamental, immutable principles such as the true, spiritual nature of a person.

Heki or 癖 generally means "a habit or inclination." Today, this kanji typically connotes a bad habit, vice, or kink. For this reason, in modern Japanese *sei heki* usually implies a negative or deviant behavior, often sexual in nature. Alternate translations might include:

- unwanted habit[1]
- innate tendency
- habit of the true self

- natural inclination
- bad habit that inhibits the expression of the true nature

This symbol is used as a tool to facilitate healing at the mental and emotional levels of being; it treats the *kokoro* directly. Its energy is decidedly softer than that of the *choku rei,* and it restores harmony any place where one is out of balance.

ORIGINS

The mental-emotional symbol, also called the "harmony symbol" in some branches of Japanese Reiki, is derived from a Sanskrit character, referred to as a seed syllable or *bonji** (梵字, "Buddhist character") in Japanese. Pronounced *hrīḥ* (which sounds rather like *hreeh*) in Sanskrit, and *kiiriku* (キリーク) in Japanese, this character is a powerful seed syllable related to the state of peace and enlightenment. Usui adapted a common seed syllable by simplifying it for ease of use. The original character that served as a model for the Reiki *shirushi* is widespread in Japan and other parts of Asia even today. It is especially common in Buddhist cemeteries and Jōdo temples throughout Japan.

Traditionally, the *hrīḥ* is found written in a script called *siddham.* These characters developed in India and are representative of sacred teachings. (The authors of Vedic texts considered their writing "divine, inherently holy, with the powers to teach the highest mysteries."[2]) The word *siddham* comes from the root *sidh,* which means "accomplished, successful, perfected, with the connotation of being sacred."[3] To the ancients, the *siddham* letters were considered uncreated. They exist according to natural principles and therefore are learned through insight.[4] This sounds like the story of Usui's revelation of the sym-

---

*In his book *This Is Reiki* (262–63), Frank Arjava Petter records an interview with Ogawa Fumio, a Reiki practitioner in Japan whose father learned Reiki Ryōhō directly from Usui-sensei. In this interview, Ogawa-san is asked about the origins of the three symbols, and he states that the second is a *bonji.*

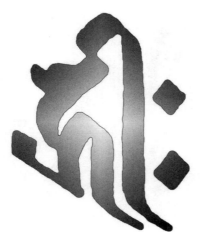

The Sanskrit seed syllable *hrīḥ*,
which is associated with peace and enlightenment

bols during his satori experience on Mount Kurama as it was told by
Hawayo Takata.

The syllable is comprised of four elements: *ha, ra, ī,* and *ḥ.*[5] Each
component corresponds to a different aspect of its meaning.

- *Ha* is the causal or karmic level of our existence. It refers to the
  part of us that exists independent of cause and therefore helps us
  restore the harmony that exists before we generate karma.
- *Ra* is the heavenly fire that offers purification. Negatively
  expressed, this fire can be our vices.
- *Ī* is the inseparability of our true nature, our own heart. When we
  buy into the illusion of separation, *ī* becomes calamity.
- *Ḥ* is the breath of life that removes negative forces and attachments. It sets us on the path to authentic liberation.

Together, these separate sounds create the *hrīḥ.* They may be interpreted as "release and salvation from all suffering."[6] The *hrīḥ* symbol,
and therefore the *sei heki* modeled on it, represents the Buddha Amida
Nyōrai (or Amitabha in Sanskrit) because it epitomizes Amida's vow to

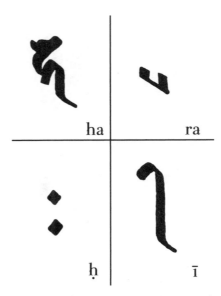

ha	ra
ḥ	ī

The *hrīḥ* is comprised of the phonetic elements *ha, ra, ī,* and *ḥ* (pictured clockwise from top left).

free all his followers from all evils.[7] In Buddhism, Amida is the central figure in the Pure Land sect (Jōdo Shū), to which Reiki founder Usui Mikao belonged. Amida is the Buddha of Boundless Light*; he is one of the five transcendental or celestial Buddhas.

Amida is regarded as the Buddha of Enlightenment and is a supreme force honored and recognized in Jōdo Buddhism. His Pure Land is the Western Paradise, associated with the archetype of bliss.[8] Reaching the Pure Land to which we aspire after complete enlightenment, however, is a one-way street; once there we are unable to return.[9] Amida acts through compassion to erase our attachments, karma, passions, and suffering so that we can find true harmony. However, since Amida dwells in the Pure Land, he cannot act directly on the human condition.

---

*Amida Nyōrai is known by many titles, including Buddha of Boundless (or Infinite) Light, Buddha of Infinite Life, Buddha of Boundless Light and Consciousness, and Buddha of Boundless Light and Life. Because of his association with unending light and his residence in the Pure Land, Amida is also considered to be the Buddha of Enlightenment.

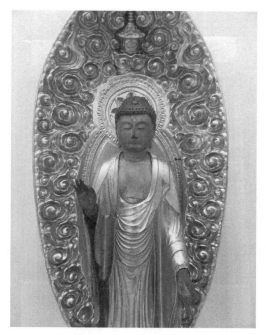

A statue of Amida Nōrai, the central figure in Jōdo Buddhism.
You may recognize the swirling motif of auspicious clouds
from our discussion in chapter 15.
Collection of George Walter Vincent Smith Art Museum

Just as Reiki is the form of ki that acts on behalf of the divine ki, or *shinki,* Amida created an intercessor of his own. Amida Nyōrai shed a tear of compassion upon recognizing the suffering of all sentient beings, and from this tear was born a special emanation of the Bodhisattva Kannon, also known as *Kuan Yin* in Chinese and *Avalokiteshvara* in Sanskrit.* Kannon is the Bodhisattva of Compassion whose name means

---

*Senju Kannon is not the only bodhisattva to be born from a tear. In Tibetan Buddhism (also called the Vajrayana or "diamond vehicle"), the Bodhisattva Tara is said to have sprung forth from the tear of Chenrezig, the Tibetan name for Avalokiteshvara or Kannon. That tear is said to have created a lake where it fell, and Tara emerged from a single lotus that blossomed in the center of the lake. Tara represents the female aspect of Chenrezig, and she is often linked to the feminine depictions of Kannon or Kuan Yin. It is possible that this Tibetan story serves as the template for the Japanese version of Senju Kannon's birth from Amida Nyōrai's tear.

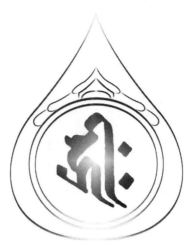

This is Amida's tear, which carries the *bonji hrīḥ.*

"one who hears the cries of the world." Bodhisattvas are in some ways analogous to saints; they are beings who have taken the bodhisattva vow, which entails forgoing total enlightenment, or entrance to the Pure Land, until every sentient being reaches that point.

This tear-shaped motif is also likened to the *cintāmaṇi* (如意宝珠 or *nyoi hōju* in Japanese), or the "wish-fulfilling jewel."[10] In many of her emanations, the Bodhisattva Kannon is depicted with this sacred stone clutched in one or both hands. Like Amida's tear, the *cintāmaṇi* is also said to have fallen from the sky, and it can confer healing or grant any wish. Since this motif often accompanies the *bonji hrīḥ* in Japanese iconography, one can infer that the *bonji* itself must embody the qualities of the *cintāmaṇi*. Thus, even the *shirushi* used in Reiki Ryōhō conveys the ability to fulfill wishes and offer deep healing. The *sei heki* is used for mental/emotional treatments, such as releasing bad habits, instilling harmony, and empowering affirmations.

The *hrīḥ* seed syllable is specifically related to a special emanation of Kannon, called the one-thousand-armed Kannon or Senju Kannon. In each of her thousand hands she carries a different tool or implement; each and every one leads us closer to enlightenment. She is invoked in some esoteric Buddhist rituals for the prevention of disease.[11] As we

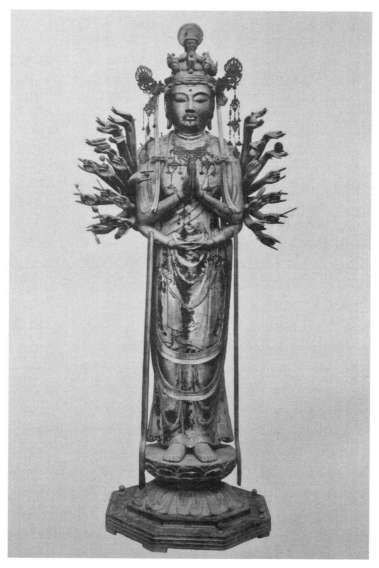

Senju Kannon, the one-thousand-armed Kuan Yin
Nara National Museum

have established, illness typically begins in the emotional or mental patterns, so use of the *sei heki* to heal the heart-mind is the key to total health. This mirrors Usui's belief about healing that when we heal the mind or *kokoro,* the body naturally returns to a state of balance.

When we use the *sei heki* symbol we are invoking the energies of infinite light and compassion, the predominant qualities of the divine beings represented by *hrīḥ*. Although the origins of the symbol are Buddhist, by simplifying the Sanskrit character and its teachings Usui made it available to everyone, no matter one's spiritual background.

The name *sei heki* is not in use in Japan in the same manner as in the West. To the common person, simply saying *sei heki* would be construed as inappropriate, for its current connotation is of a sexual nature. However, the expression *sei heki* is a shortened name of the therapy that employs the harmony symbol: *sei heki chiryō* (性癖治療). Translated into English, it means "treatment of bad habits" or "healing method for bad habits." Jikiden Reiki properly calls it *sei heki no shirushi* (性癖の印, "bad habit symbol")[12] or *sei heki chiryō no shirushi* (性癖治療の印, "symbol of treating bad habits").

The original method for using the *sei heki* made use of a sacred invocation or *kotodama* that commanded the true self to correct the named bad habit. When Hawayo Takata began to teach people who didn't speak Japanese, she made a conscious choice to simplify the protocol in using this symbol for treatment. Researcher and practitioner Jojan Jonker notes that "the Japanese incantation probably sounded like abracadabra for native English speakers, just like the word *seiheki* itself. Thus, the ritual got simplified; the word *sei heki* replaced the incantation and afterwards became a sacred and secret mantra."[13]

Similar to the manner in which the original *kotodama* identifies the bad habit, reciting the phrase *sei heki* calls out to whichever bad habit is in need of resolution, thereby imploring the recipient's true, spiritual nature to address the negative pattern in order to return to wholeness. Although the connotation of the phrase *sei heki* has changed over time in Japan, the essential meaning of the kanji themselves invokes the original nature of our *kokoro*. Thus, when we speak this mantra aloud, the *kotodama,* or soul of these words, loosens and transmutes any habits that inhibit the heart's truest and healthiest expression.

THE HARMONIOUS QUALITIES OF *SEI HEKI*

The second *shirushi* is referred to as the harmony symbol in some schools of Reiki Ryōhō in Japan; it is meant to instill peace and harmony in our heart-minds. It is the symbol that works directly upon the *kokoro,* and its primary action is to heal opposing forces. Even the outer shape of the *sei heki* resembles two opposing factions; the harmony symbol is the mediating force between the dual natures of our existence.

Connecting to the *sei heki* awakens a knowing of the true self by releasing attachment to duality and the material world. Attachment to the world around us is the cause of much of our suffering, and so it is that the harmony symbol gently and compassionately brings our attention to the real nature of our *kokoro.* It's a mirror that reflects our divine template for peace and success in all things. When we arrive at this awareness of self we can stop grasping at the material world. This, in turn, prevents both attachment and the formation of bad habits.

Whenever the *sei heki* is drawn, its energy brings Reiki to the causal point (*ha*) in order to purify (*ra*) the heart (*i*) with the breath of life (*h*). The *sei heki* becomes a mediating force that purifies and detaches the awareness from the material plane and the illusion of separation. As it releases duality's hold over the psyche, the heart and mind return to their original state of unity with one another and with the divine mind. In this way the harmony symbol also erases the karmic effects of our decisions and habits to pave the way to *anshin ritsumei.*

USING *SEI HEKI*

Traditionally, the *sei heki* has a single indication in *dento Reiki,* which is the *sei heki chiryō,* or treatment of bad habits. Because the original invocation or *kotodama* employed in this technique is kept secret, some additional methods will also be described for using the harmony symbol. This *shirushi* can be drawn over yourself or your client whenever there is a condition rooted in the emotions or mental patterns. Its action reaches deep into the subconscious to uproot hidden traumas or other psychological conditions.

The effect of using the second *shirushi* is one of overall release. It alleviates stress, soothes unbalanced emotions, breaks repetitive habits and thoughts, and cuts energetic cords. It can be used in techniques that reprogram the mind via affirmations, such as the Japanese technique *nentatsu hō,* and it also makes an excellent adjunct to reciting the *gokai.* The *sei heki* can also be drawn on parts of the body suffering from physical conditions that result from emotional or mental patterns, such as psychosomatic illness or conditions left over from karmic energies.

Whenever anger, worry, stress, fear, anxiety, or other strong emotions are impacting you or your client, the harmony symbol can be invoked to mitigate them. This symbol is extremely nourishing and it helps one overcome negative patterns in relatively short time. Regular use of this symbol can radically change perceptions, feelings, and actions for the better. Use the *sei heki* for:

- stress and stress-related illness
- confusion
- sadness, sorrow, and anguish
- forgiveness
- low self-esteem
- eating disorders
- dementia
- violence
- depression and anxiety
- isolationism
- phobias
- panic disorder

Given that the primary application of the *sei heki* is in altering our habits, it's best applied consciously with a specific outcome in mind. It can be drawn while you meditate on the desired result or before you begin to recite an affirmation or prayer. Drawing it over a part of the body with the intent to release trapped emotional energy is also effective.

Some additional uses for the mental-emotional *shirushi* mostly derived from Western Reiki branches include:

- instilling group harmony; it can be used for small groups, communities, or nations
- improving sleep
- improving memory
- finding lost objects
- correcting behavioral challenges in pets
- cultivating equanimity and compassion
- generating loving thoughts
- manifesting world peace
- repairing bone, muscle, and visceral conditions via *sei heki chiryō*[14]

In addition to the following exercises, chapter 18 on *okuden* Japanese Reiki Techniques includes methods for using the *sei heki* in healing.

❖ Empowering Affirmations

Because the second *shirushi* acts to help us correct our habits, it's highly effective when combined with affirmations. Select a new behavior or mental pattern that you'd like to learn and integrate; write it down on a piece of paper and use this technique to enhance your results.

1. Write your affirmation or prayer on a note card. It should be phrased in the present tense and articulated as a positive outcome.
2. Place the card between your hands in *gasshō* and spend a few moments connecting to the flow of Reiki.
3. Using your entire hand, draw the *sei heki* in the air above the note card; recite its name and tap the card three times.
4. Hold your affirmation card in your hands and give it Reiki while reciting your affirmation aloud or in your mind. If you desire, draw the *choku rei* afterward to amplify and ground the effects of the harmony symbol.

5. Carry your card with you and periodically give it Reiki while reciting the affirmation like a mantra.

6. Repeat this process daily until your new habit has manifested.

❖ Treating Psychogenic Conditions

Originating in the practice of Kōmyō Reiki Dō, this is a simple treatment for psychogenic and psychosomatic conditions.[15] Because the second *shirushi* heals disharmony and karmic patterns that reside in the mental and emotional levels, it can be employed to treat conditions with physical manifestations that result from the psychological level. Combining the psychological treatment with traditional hands-on healing will enable practitioners to use a well-rounded approach.

1. Draw the *sei heki* on each of the temples of the head.

2. Place your hands on the temples and treat them with Reiki. Treat for at least one full cycle of *byōsen,* or until it dissipates altogether.

3. Draw the *shirushi* on the stomach.

4. Treat the stomach with both hands for at least one full cycle of *byōsen.*

5. Treat the areas in which symptoms are present, if they remain. Follow normal treatment methods.

❖ Deprogramming Technique

Usui Shiki Reiki Ryōhō preserves the *sei heki chiryō* methods in a slightly modified format as a treatment usually referred to as the deprogramming technique. It makes use of the first two *shirushi:* the *choku rei* and the *sei heki.* The steps are remarkably similar to *nentatsu hō* (see chapter 18), aside from the use of an additional *shirushi.* Though there are several extant versions of the deprogramming treatment, I have elected to use the style presented by authors Walter Lübeck and Frank Arjava Petter in *Reiki Best Practices.*[16] Though described below as if treating a client, this exercise can easily be used on oneself.

1. Begin by writing a short affirmation that encapsulates the goal of the treatment; it may be written by practitioner and client together, or soley by the client. Ensure that the affirmation is positive, with no mention of illness or disharmony.

2. Draw the *choku rei* on the back of the client's head with one hand; silently repeat its name three times. Continue to hold your hand over the back of the head and allow Reiki to flow.

3. Draw the *sei heki* over the base of the skull (where the medulla oblongata is located). Repeat its name silently three times.

4. Draw the *choku rei* over the base of the skull and silently repeat its name three times.

5. Keeping one hand over the base of the skull, place the other over your client's forehead. Repeat the chosen affirmation three times either silently or aloud. Ask the client to do the same, with as much sincerity and intensity as he or she can muster. At this point I usually continue to treat the client silently for several minutes.

6. Gently remove your hands from the client when the treatment is complete. Consider a self-cleansing *gihō* such as *kenyoku hō* after the treatment.

In the following chapter we will move on to discuss the third symbol: *hon sha ze shō nen*. This is an exciting, dynamic symbol in that it is primarily used when treating from a distance, making one's reach as a practitioner of Reiki that much greater.

17

THE THIRD SYMBOL:
HON SHA ZE SHŌ NEN

UNLIKE THE PREVIOUS TWO SYMBOLS, *hon sha ze shō nen* (abbreviated *HSZSN*) is considered a *jumon* rather than *shirushi*. Used in remote or absentee healing, this *jumon* is often simply called the distance symbol or the connection symbol. It is constructed from five kanji; the overlapping characters have the repeated radicals omitted in order to stack them together in a simplified, encoded form. *Hon sha ze shō nen* is composed of the following five characters: 本者是正念. Each of these signs has multiple meanings in Japanese, as well as in their original Chinese contexts.

Hon, or 本, typically means "book," "this," "basis," "origin," "source," or "foundation." It is also used as a counter for cylindrical objects in the Japanese language. *Sha,* 者, is a person. Rather than represent humankind generally, it is often used to indicate a person engaged in a specific activity, or else for emphasis.[1] In this way it has a commanding tone.[2] *Ze,* written 是, can mean "right" or "just," but in this case it retains its original use in Chinese as the verb "to be." *Shō,* 正, can mean "correct," "adjust," "agreement," "proper goal," or "this." Finally, *nen* (念) can mean "sense," "feeling," "thought," or "desire." Note the *kokoro* radical (心) at its base.

When we put these five words together they form a sentence.

Although the predominant pronunciation of this *jumon* is *hon sha ze shō nen*, several alternate pronunciations are extant in Japan; each character has more than one reading, so there is a lack of agreement on this point among some practitioners today. The meanings of these characters are multidimensional, and thus there are many different levels of interpretations available. Some may include:

- Origin of man is right mind (mindfulness).
- This person is right mind.
- The root of everything is right consciousness.[3]
- The basics to become happy start with right consciousness.[4]
- I am right mind.[5]
- My original self is correct thought.[6]
- The Buddha in me meets the Buddha in you.[7]

Although each translation differs from the others, sometimes in very subtly nuanced ways, we see that these five syllables contain a treasury of ideas. The *HSZSN* symbol is conveying a truly esoteric matter. Reiki *shihan* and author Frans Stiene describes this in his book *The Inner Heart of Reiki* when he writes: "In looking at the translation of this mantra we can already see that it has nothing to do with distance healing. In fact the opposite is true; it is about rediscovering that there is no distance at all!"[8]

ORIGINS

The *jumon* used for distance healing is an original invention of Usui-sensei. If one were to share the symbol itself with a native speaker of Japanese or Chinese, the characters would not be clearly understood because of their overlap. Usui-sensei designed this motif after his rigorous spiritual studies and subsequent revelation or awakening on Mount Kurama. The choice of words, however, may point us toward his sources of inspiration.

The final character of *HSZSN* on its own, *nen* or 念, has a wide range of associations. It is a combination of the characters for *now* and *heart:* 今 and 心. Most of the possible translations of *nen* take us into an understanding that it is reflecting what our heart-mind (*kokoro*) is focused on, such as hopes, desires, wishes, thoughts, and feelings. It's literally what's in our hearts right now. *Nen* is used in a large number of compound words with spiritual associations, including the words for prayer beads and an expression for reciting magical formulas.

The last two characters of *HSZSN* are a special term in Buddhism. *Shōnen* or 正念 means "mindfulness," "right mind," or even "Buddha Consciousness." Usui may have looked into the esoteric principles of some branches of Buddhism in order to borrow this expression for its spiritual value and the vibration of its *kotodama.* Right mind or right mindfulness is even one of the aspects of the Eightfold Path of Buddhism.* *Shōnen* can also be taken to mean "mentally healthy" outside of its spiritual context.[9] In light of this, Usui chose this phrase to remind his students that healing the mind comes first.

The overall shape of the distance healing *jumon* is reminiscent of a Taoist method of preparing ritual charms and talismans; the characters can be stacked or superimposed so as to be illegible to the layperson.[10] This procedure is surprisingly similar to the creation of bind runes, sacred symbols with talismanic properties derived from early Germanic writing systems. Usui is known to have applied himself to many different paths of spiritual lore, making a Taoist connection not unlikely.

These Taoist charms or talismans are referred to as *fuwen* (符文) in Chinese, and they are magical or talismanic writing. The inscriptions have been used as spells for a multitude of purposes throughout history. Talismanic calligraphy has long been employed as a means of connecting with the supernatural or mystical realms. Those of a Buddhist variety

---

*One Japanese branch of Reiki in particular makes use of an alternate reading of these two characters, thereby circumventing the overtly religious connotation that *shōnen* has in Japan today. Usui developed his Reiki Ryōhō to be nonreligious so that it could be accessible to people of any background. However, I have not yet found sufficient evidence to definitively state whether Usui used the Buddhist reading of these kanji or a more secular pronunciation.

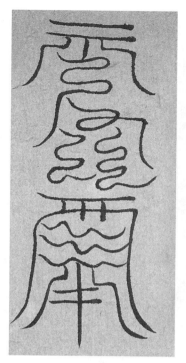 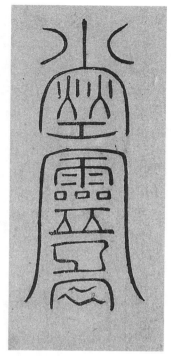

Here are two examples of Chinese calligraphic talismans. Both are used for healing. The one pictured on the right contains the character 靈 (*ling* in Chinese and *rei* in Japanese), meaning "soul" or "spirit," as in *Reiki*.

Wellcome Library

may even incorporate Sanskrit seed syllables, a practice that continues in China and Japan today.[11] Many of the surviving *fuwen* are for healing, although they are typically written on paper or leaves, unlike the long-distance healing *jumon*, which traditionally was never written down.

Similar uses of writing kanji in close contact with one another can be found in styles of one-line calligraphy and in the calligraphic mandalas of Nichiren Buddhism. Descended from the Taoist *fuwen* charms, these examples of sacred writing superficially resemble the style used to create the *HSZSN*. There are cases when the individual characters begin to overlap enough to make it difficult to decipher the meaning of the inscription. Master calligraphers seek to capture the ki with their brushes; they are creating visible renderings of the *kotodama*, or the soul

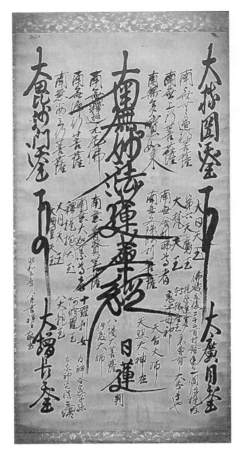

The *gohonzon,* a mandala of calligraphic formula venerated in Nichiren Buddhism in Japan. The overlapping kanji and Sanskrit seed syllables are reminiscent of the shape and style of the distance healing *jumon.*

Calligraphy from the author's collection, photo by Steven Thomas Walsh

of their words. Perhaps Usui Mikao accomplished something similar when he crafted this *jumon.*

Some researchers have attempted to make tenuous connections between the five characters of the *HSZSN* and the five elements, the cardinal directions, and various other correspondences. These connections are generally unlikely; the words were probably chosen for the strength of their *kotodama,* which would serve as fuel for a *jumon* or incantation.

One last interesting association is offered by writers and Reiki teachers Walter Lübeck and Mark Hosak, who discuss the similarities between the shape of the *HSZSN* and the classical form of the pagoda with its upturned eaves.[12] The pagoda itself is inspired by the stupa, a dome-like monument or reliquary often topped by a pointed spire. Stupas originated as markers of sacred sites in Buddhist cultures. The central column or pillar that supports the pagoda is called the *shinhashira* or heart pillar (心柱). Typically, relics or sacred texts are stored beneath the heart pillar; they are the "objects that, simply expressed, make sure that the Buddha and his energy—meaning the 'Buddha Consciousness'—are present."[13] This Buddha Consciousness is an interpretation of *shōnen,* whose second character (念) ends with the symbol for heart, or *kokoro.* This kanji is the metaphorical heart pillar upon which the form of the *HSZSN* is built.

QUALITIES OF CONNECTION

Japanese branches of Reiki sometimes call the *HSZSN* the connection symbol, rather than the distance healing symbol as Western lineages typically do. This is likely due in part to the Western mind's desire to separate and catalog experiences, whereas the Japanese perspective celebrates unity and inclusion. The *HSZSN* was created to work in this way; it acts upon the part of the mind in which there is no separation, and therefore no distance.

The translations of the *jumon* point toward the origins or roots of the human experience. *HSZSN* is a tool that guides the practitioner's awareness to the primordial spark from which we all come. It takes us to a place before illness, before unhappiness, before separation. This spark contains the perfect blueprint for happiness, success, and perfect health. At this level of existence, neither time nor distance exists. Everything is one.

Several of the translations of *shōnen* listed above describe it as being related to something holy and perfected, such as Buddha Consciousness, God, or the original essence of humankind. The divine nature of reality knows no boundaries, however. This is how the *HSZSN* works; it affects us where there is no distance. Hosak and Lübeck write that "time and space are not boundaries for the Buddha Consciousness—it exists in every being as a potential and can be awakened to life through the right means."[14]

Whenever the connection *jumon* is drawn and recited, it transcends the perceived distance between practitioner and recipient. This allows us to share Reiki with anyone, anywhere in the world, at any time. We can use this symbol to heal someone who is miles away just as easily as we can heal someone by a laying on of hands. This *jumon* can also be used to send healing forward and backward in time.

The esoteric mechanism at work is not literally sending Reiki, however. Instead, when the practitioner writes the *HSZSN* and speaks its name aloud, the receiver and the practitioner come together as one. Although we speak of "sending" Reiki in remote treatments, we are calling that soul spark of the client to the practitioner where it joins with the practitioner on the level of pure consciousness. This is one of the limitations of describing something as ineffable as Reiki in words. It might be more accurate to tell a client or a friend that you'll be connecting with them on the soul level to share Reiki with them in a space where time and space are absent, but doing so would probably elicit a puzzled stare from them.

Because the symbol invokes the original consciousness, which exists outside of linear time, we can pinpoint any event in the past or future and offer it Reiki. Although Usui and Hayashi never taught techniques like this, the possibility of applying the *HSZSN* for healing across time is no less real than transcending physical distance. This symbol is also a powerful tool for releasing the memory of trauma; it can easily be combined with the *sei heki* to do so. As well, it's an effective tool for preparing for an upcoming event of any type; simply use the symbol to project Reiki forward to the moment when it will be needed.

USING *HON SHA ZE SHŌ NEN*

The practical applications of the distance healing *jumon* are many and varied. Its primary function is to eliminate the perceived distance between the practitioner and recipient; Reiki is omnipresent, so it is not bound by physical distance. Whenever we invoke this *jumon* we are bringing our client into our heart-mind to be one with us in Reiki. Using the *HSZSN* allows us to practice Reiki without limitations.

The connection symbol is a valuable tool for practitioners because it allows the practitioner to treat family, friends, and clients without them being physically present. Use it to connect to clients before and after they arrive for in-person sessions or as a means of sending your loving intentions to your family, no matter where they are. You may also use it in tandem with the two *shirushi* to target *byōsen* and to offer support for emotional or mental healing.

To use the symbol most effectively, gather as much information about the recipient as possible. In order to connect with him or her effectively, it helps to have the person's full name and date of birth. A photo of the client or description of the condition being treated is also beneficial. If the personal information about the recipient of Reiki is unknown, simply connect to Reiki and ask that it be directed where needed.

Some anecdotal evidence concerning the development of remote treatments in Reiki Ryōhō has been shared by Doi Hiroshi. Usui's methods apparently developed over time to accommodate students of different educational, social, and economic backgrounds. At the onset, Usui-sensei's students were encouraged to use photographs of their clients for distance healing (see *shashin chiryō hō* on page 273), but this was an expense that not everyone could afford. Over time, photographs were substituted with drawings of the clients (perhaps labeled with names and other personal information). In the end, "practitioners and teachers realized that a physical image is not necessary at all to successfully send distant healing."[15]

In modern styles of Reiki Ryōhō, a symbol is drawn and its mantra is repeated three times to activate its healing power. Remember that *shirushi* such as the first two Reiki symbols do not require a mantra to work; however, as the connection symbol is really a *jumon,* its *kotodama* fuels its effects. The *HSZSN* may be drawn in the air as you visualize the person, over a photo or note card with the recipient's name and personal information on it, on a surrogate like a pillow or teddy bear, or over a part of your own body standing in for the client. You can then treat as normal, especially noting the sensations of *byōsen*.

When doing this, it's nearly always more effective to treat one person at a time, as you can sense and respond to the *byōsen* that arises. Treating multiple people, large groups, or nonliving targets (such as a place, situation, region, or the like) will not yield the sensations of *byōsen* in a manner that can be effectively treated in real time. Although it is possible to send healing in such circumstances, the effects may be more diluted than if the practitioner focuses on a single person. The technique taught by Hayashi-sensei, called *enkaku chiryō*, enables practitioners to treat two people simultaneously. In Japan, distance healing was only used for treating human beings in Usui Reiki Ryōhō; any other applications are the result of more recent innovations.

In sending Reiki to past events, the distance healing *jumon* is used to release any connection or underlying trauma. Try to obtain a photo from the time frame to which you'd like to send Reiki; otherwise, just conjure the image of the event in your mind. For easing its emotional aftermath, combine *HSZSN* with the *sei heki* symbol. This technique can be applied to impersonal scenarios too, such as sending Reiki to a group, place, or time affected by trauma.

To prepare for future events, the connection *jumon* can help the practitioner send Reiki ahead in time, also. Inwardly choose the point at which you or your client would like to receive a boost of Reiki and draw and recite the *jumon*. This technique is great for interviews, meetings, tests, performances, medical procedures, and other scheduled events. Performance during the appointed time is usually enhanced, with many people reporting greater calm and focus with this application.

During a hands-on session, the distance healing *jumon* also deepens the connection between practitioner and recipient. It can facilitate deeper healing by directing Reiki into the cause, especially when it is unknown. In these cases, *HSZSN* acts like a homing device that can tap into Reiki's innate intelligence to reach core issues. When the *jumon* is used with this intention, it will seek out the *byōgen* in order to treat it at the most fundamental level. The practitioner can thus target the cause of illnesses or injuries that present with complex or confusing *byōsen* patterns in order to resolve them from the ground up.

APPLICATIONS

- To send healing when separated by distance
- To treat part of your own body that you can't reach, such as your own back
- To send Reiki forward and backward in time
- To prepare a client before a session
- To follow up with your clients in between sessions
- As a homing device when the underlying cause is unknown
- To heal the underlying karmic energy of an illness or other condition
- To find lost objects
- To scan a client, object, or place remotely, such as via *reiji hō* and *byōsen reikan hō*

ABOUT PERMISSION

Permission is a derisive topic among many practitioners of healing modalities. In Reiki, I was initially taught that permission must *always* be granted before proceeding to send distance Reiki. In the event that the recipient is unable to outright ask for or consent to Reiki, such as when treating infants, sleeping or comatose persons, or other individuals, the practitioner can rely on his or her inner guidance to determine whether or not the higher self of the client is willing to receive Reiki. In these instances, seldom is it refused.

However, from a Japanese point of view permission is generally regarded as unnecessary. Usui-sensei has said that Reiki works independently of belief in or knowledge of its use; he indicates that recipients benefit whether they are skeptics or believers or are aware of it being sent. In general, lineages of Japanese Reiki affirm that since we are all connected (which is the real message behind *hon sha ze shō nen*), we have a right and duty to offer healing. To heal one person, even oneself, is to heal all of humankind.

As we know, Reiki never causes harm, has no contraindications, and is a gentle therapy meant to uplift and heal all people. There is no harm in sending Reiki in emergency situations, when someone does not understand Reiki or energy healing, or when the recipient cannot speak or communicate. Wherever possible, it's best to involve clients in their own health and happiness. If someone consents to receive Reiki, it can signal to his or her subconscious a true desire to get well.

And although Reiki can always help, it may not solve every condition. In these instances Reiki can offer compassionate palliative care.

❈ Distance Healing

In general, there are many ways to apply the connection symbol. For starters, collect information about your recipient so you may connect more deeply. If a photo is unavailable, you can choose to write his or her name and personal information on a piece of paper. Start with sending distance Reiki to one recipient at a time so as not to diffuse its effects.

1. Begin with the photo or piece of paper with your client's information on it. Draw the *jumon* in the air above it and recite *hon sha ze shō nen* three times.

2. Visualize the person between your hands or hold the photo/card between your hands. Allow Reiki to flow to the recipient as you picture him or her.

3. Proceed with a normal treatment, paying attention to *byōsen*; use the *choku rei* as necessary. For psychological treatments, use the *sei heki*.

4. When you're ready to conclude your treatment, simply stop sending Reiki.

❈ Healing with a Surrogate

If you are uncomfortable visualizing or would prefer to simulate hands-on Reiki sessions, try using a pillow or stuffed animal as a stand-in for the client. This way, you can treat each individual area of the client's body just as you would face-to-face.

1. Collect your client's personal information, as before, and prepare yourself for Reiki. You may cleanse your surrogate, such as by using *jaki kiri jōka hō* (see chapter 18).

2. Set your intention to connect to the recipient and pray for or focus on his or her healing.

3. Draw the *HSZSN* in the air over the surrogate; recite the mantra three times.

4. Treat just as you would if the client were with you in person.

❖ Sending Reiki to the Past or Future

One of the most life-changing techniques that I learned in my first Reiki classes was how to use the connection *jumon* to bridge time. You can use either of the former healing techniques if you are sending Reiki to another person (or even to yourself), although you can visualize the outcome just as well. Refine the time frame as specifically as possible and follow the directions below.

1. Connect as before using whichever tools or props you have available. Set your intention to send Reiki into the past or future.

2. Draw the symbol in the air in front of you and recite the mantra for *HSZSN* three times.

3. Visualize sending Reiki to the desired point in time. If you are healing the past, combine it with the necessary *shirushi* to tackle whichever remnants of the trauma you encounter.

4. When you are finished sending Reiki, close with the *choku rei* to seal the process and anchor the positive changes. Express your gratitude for the blessings that Reiki brings.

For more exercises in distance healing, please see the Japanese Reiki Techniques in the following chapter.

18

MORE JAPANESE REIKI TECHNIQUES

SEVERAL HELPFUL TECHNIQUES from Japan were introduced in the *shoden* level. These tools empower practitioners to strengthen the flow of Reiki, enhance and ground their meditative practices, and apply specialized methods of hands-on healing with Reiki. The following *Nihon no Reiki gihō* (Japanese Reiki Techniques) help Reiki practitioners grow further in their self-development and in offering themselves in service to others through Reiki.

Any of the previously discussed tools can be enhanced by the use of the *shirushi* and *jumon,* although this combination of tools may not be the standard practice in Japan. *Koki hō* and *gyōshi hō* are especially effective when combined with the symbols; additional instructions will be included below. Traditional methods of mental-emotional healing and absentee healing are also included in this list; they may be used in tandem with or in lieu of Western methods for the same outcomes.

Finally, the *gihō* that fall under the heading of *hatsurei hō* are among the most important tools for practitioners who seek personal development and spiritual growth through Reiki. Engaging in these practices will strengthen your connection to Reiki, as well as to your higher self, facilitating greater healing within and without. Each of the *hatsurei hō* techniques was introduced by Usui-sensei as a means of helping his students develop a sense of *anshin ritsumei.* Practicing them on your own can foster a greater sense of peace, better health, and a deeper spiritual connection to the world.

❈ *Gyōshi Hō* and *Koki Hō* Revisited

My first introduction to these two healing methods employed the *okuden* symbols. When I later revisited Reiki from a more Japanese perspective, the idea of using the symbols with the breath or gaze was entirely absent. However, because these methods work so well, I encourage you to try out these Western adaptations of traditional techniques.

Koki hō can be combined with the first *shirushi* in order to concentrate the power of Reiki onto a single locus. Doing so breaks up stagnant energy, blockages, and disharmony. It is one of my favorite means of targeting strong *byōsen.* Wait to use it until you feel the crest of the cycle. The sensations should then immediately return to the lowest degree, thus beginning the next cycle. Use a single pulsed exhale, rather than the long focused breath. You may also try *koki hō* with the other symbols to reach psychological patterns or to dig into and resolve karmic energies at work.

By drawing the distance healing *jumon* before engaging in *gyōshi hō,* practitioners can connect with the many levels of a client's existence. Then, sending Reiki with the eyes becomes an experience in seeing beyond the physical body. Many practitioners report flashes of past lives or memories of trauma; they may even see symbols related to their clients' spiritual growth. Although this is a Westernized approach, combining *HSZSN* with *gyōshi hō* is extremely powerful.

Koki Hō Instructions

1. Draw the *choku rei* or *sei heki* on the roof of your mouth with your tongue; silently recite the mantra three times. (If using the third symbol, drawing it may be uncomfortable or difficult; in this case, simply visualize the *jumon* in your mouth.)
2. Bring the tip of your tongue to the roof of your mouth and inhale deeply and fully. Briefly pause and focus on the chosen *shirushi* or *jumon.*
3. Exhale through the mouth in a short, quick burst of air. If practicing this

during hands-on treatment, such as to neutralize *byōsen,* gently pivot or lift your hands from the client's body on the exhale and return them immediately thereafter.

Gyōshi Hō Instructions

1. With your client seated or reclined, encourage him or her to close the eyes and relax completely.

2. Draw the *HSZSN* in the air between you and your client. Set your intention to connect to Reiki in order to send it with your eyes.

3. Relax your gaze and direct your attention to your client. Allow your eyes to defocus.

4. Continue sending Reiki with your eyes; your gaze may be drawn to a particular area or move from one area to another. As you are treating, acknowledge any images, sensations, or symbols that arise.

5. When you are finished, draw the *choku rei* in the air over the client. You may now end the session or continue with hands-on treatment.

6. Afterward, discuss any relevant messages or symbols that came through. Invite your client to meditate on these and to integrate the healing that they offer.

❖ *Jaki Kiri Jōka Hō* 邪氣切り浄化法

Jaki kiri jōka hō is a method of using Reiki to cleanse or clear an object's energy. Its name literally translates as "method for purification by cutting negative energy." It is a simple way of purifying crystals, gifts, healing tools, and other objects without any additional props. It should be used only on inanimate objects; use other healing or meditative Reiki techniques for purifying people or other living things.[1]

Once connected to Reiki, the practitioner holds the selected object in his or her nondominant hand and proceeds with the physical motions of *jaki kiri jōka hō*. In instances where the object is too large to hold, it can be placed on the floor before you, or you can "do it via distant healing or with a photograph of the object."[2] It can be used on hotel beds, on massage tables before and after treatments, or even on buildings and houses as a means of clearing disharmonious or negative energy.

1. Begin in *gasshō* and connect to Reiki.
2. Place the object in your nondominant hand and draw in the breath. Breathe all the way into your lower *tanden,* imagining it filling with Reiki energy.
3. With your dominant hand, cut or chop the air horizontally, two to three inches above the object while holding the breath. In total, make approximately three cutting movements; use more or less as you intuitively feel guided to do. Stop the movement abruptly after the last chop.
4. Release the breath and give the object Reiki while breathing normally.
5. Repeat as needed. Some items may require two or more applications of *jaki kiri jōka hō.*

❖ *Hatsurei Hō* 發靈法

In forming Reiki Ryōhō, founder Usui Mikao developed a group of techniques that, when practiced together, are collectively known as *hatsurei hō.* Their aim is to enhance the practitioner's relationship to Reiki. *Hatsurei hō* literally means "method for discharging or generating soul" or *rei[ki].* *Hatsu* means "to generate," "discharge," "leave," or "start." Now written as 発, *hatsu* or 發 has a wide array of meanings associated with it.

Different schools of Reiki Ryōhō in Japan have adapted *hatsurei hō* to suit their needs. In Jikiden Reiki and Gendai Reiki Hō the practice has been simplified to enable more practitioners to engage. The method prescribed in Jikiden's teachings covers a series of exercises over five days. Most other methods use a three-part structure, consisting of *kenyoku hō, jōshin kokyū hō,* and a version of *gasshō meiso* often referred to as *seishin tōitsu.*

Given that it's impossible to know exactly how Usui taught *hatsurei hō,* the best we can do is adopt a method that works for us or try to reconstruct his method by studying how it changed over the generations. The following three exercises closely resemble the Japanese versions from several branches of Reiki Ryōhō.

When one makes use of these meditations and exercises, sensitivity to *byōsen* will be enhanced. One may feel more energized and peaceful and bring oneself closer to *anshin ritsumei.* The best way to approach the three parts of *hatsurei hō* is to master each one in sequence; only move to the next one when it's comfortable to do so. Ideally, spending thirty minutes or more each day for five to seven days will significantly improve the ability to facilitate Reiki sessions. If that time is uncomfortable or impossible for you to schedule, start with five to ten minutes and work your way up.

The first *hatsurei hō* method is *kenyoku hō,* which is discussed in chapter 8. Please review the instructions and then proceed to the second *hatsurei hō,* called *jōshin kokyū hō.* After developing proficiency in the second technique, you may advance to the third and final part of the exercise, *seishin tōitsu.*

Jōshin Kokyū Hō 浄心呼吸法

The second *hatsurei hō* is called *jōshin kokyū hō.* Translated from Japanese, it roughly means "method for purifying the heart (*kokoro*) by breathing." *Kokyū* is a compound word comprised of the kanji for "exhale" and "inhale." *Jōshin* is "pure or clean heart," here meaning "purification of the *kokoro.*" The method uses the breath, and therefore the ki carried with it, to clear away accumulations of stagnant energy, disharmony, and self-limiting beliefs and feelings in order to refine one's vessel (the physical body) for an improved flow of Reiki.

After performing *kenyoku hō,* sit in *seiza,* or cross-legged, on the floor. Place the hands palms up on the knees or thighs; the hands should be relaxed and very slightly cupped. Once comfortable, set your intention to practice *jōshin kokyū hō* and complete the breathing exercise below. By breathing down into the *tanden,* the passageways through which Reiki naturally flows are strengthened. The recommended duration is approximately thirty minutes.

1. Perform *kenyoku.*
2. While seated, rest the hands on the legs, palms upward.
3. With each inhale, visualize light or ki flowing through the nose and down into the *shimotanden* (lower *tanden* or *hara*).
4. Between the incoming breath and outgoing breath, pause briefly and picture the concentrated energy expanding from the *hara* through the entire body. If a prevailing condition prevents you from holding the breath, visualize this expansion of energy the moment the breath turns from in to out.

5. With the exhalation expand the ki further, permitting it to extend beyond the physical body and out into the room. Let the energy course through your entire energy field, letting it expand more and more.

6. Repeat steps 3 through 5 until you are ready to finish.

7. Finish the exercise by placing the hands in *gasshō* and giving thanks.[3]

Seishin Tōitsu 精神統一

Once *jōshin kokyū hō* has become second nature, practitioners progress to the third stage of *hatsurei hō*. This technique is sometimes referred to as *gasshō kokyū hō*, or *gasshō* breathing method, a title descriptive of the outer form embodied by this technique. The name *seishin tōitsu* (精神統一) is a term used in schools of martial arts and some forms of Buddhism.

Sei (精) means "spirit," "vitality," "to refine," or "detail." It's derived from the radicals for "rice" and "blue/green," here meaning "pure." *Spirit* comes from the connotation of "freshness" and "purity." The second kanji is the same as the word *kami*, 神; together *seishin* means "spirit," with the connotation of "a refined or purified spirit." *Tōitsu* generally translates as "unity." Thus, *seishin tōitsu* is a state of unification and purification of the spirit.

In the traditional Japanese arts, *seishin tōitsu* can be accomplished through meditation, calligraphy, martial arts, flower arranging, or preparing tea. Usui-sensei taught his pupils a meditation that also yields this same state of focus and unity. After purifying one's inner vessel through the practice of *jōshin kokyū hō*, the hands are placed in *gasshō* and the breath is again harnessed for the third and final part of *hatsurei hō*. As before, one should practice this only when familiar with the earlier components of *hatsurei hō*. One should also try to devote up to thirty minutes each day with it. The more *seishin tōitsu* is practiced, the stronger the flow of Reiki will be when it's applied for hands-on healing.

1. Perform *kenyoku hō*.

2. Spend time following the above instructions for *jōshin kokyū hō*.

3. Place the hands in *gasshō* and affirm the intention to practice *seishin tōitsu*.

4. With each inhale imagine the breath and its ki being drawn in through the hands (still in *gasshō*) and down into the *tanden*.

5. On the exhale, allow the energy to reverse its flow, traveling from the

tanden through the body and out the palms of the hands. It also may be pictured flowing out the soles of the feet.

6. Repeat steps 4 and 5 until you are ready to complete the *seishin tōitsu* exercise.

7. Breathe normally with the hands still in *gasshō.* Center yourself in gratitude.

❖ *Nentatsu Hō* 念達法

Nentatsu hō is one of the original methods used for healing at the mental and emotional levels. The name is difficult to render in English concisely, but it roughly equates to "a method for reaching into the subconscious." *Nen* (念) is the final character in *hon sha ze shō nen,* the distance healing *jumon.* As previously discussed, *nen* contains the radical for the heart, *kokoro,* which will point toward the nature of this *gihō.*

The translations for *nen* are varied, and they include "strong will," "strong desire," "emotional force," "intention," "intense concentration," and "strong control by mind or consciousness."[4] In his capacity as a Reiki researcher, Doi-sensei writes that since *nen* tends to be used to satisfy ego or selfish desire, Reiki healers are taught *not* to use it while healing.[5] The second kanji, *tatsu* or 達, means "to reach," "over," "of," "up," and similar concepts. Thus, *nentatsu hō* is the method for reaching our ego-fueled forces and strong emotions in order to reconcile and reorganize them with Reiki.

The technique itself is similar to the deprogramming technique of Usui Shiki Ryōhō, although it is not necessary to use any of the symbols for *nentatsu hō.* Some lineages of Reiki have employed *nentatsu* as a means of detoxifying the mind and body, and the procedures may differ slightly among practitioners in Japan. The following method draws upon several sources for inspiration and makes use of the second *shirushi* to deepen its effect.

Nentatsu hō can be used on oneself or one's clients. It will be necessary to choose an affirmation that will guide the subconscious toward making positive change. In lieu of writing an affirmation, the *gokai* may be used. Explain to the client in advance that once the affirmations have been recited, he or she can make the most of the therapy by reflecting on or reciting the words internally for the duration of the treatment. Avoid saying anything else during this technique, as you are programming very specific intentions.

1. Begin by selecting an affirmation that supports positive growth or healing; alternatively, use the *gokai*.

2. Spend a few moments in *gasshō* and connect to Reiki. It is important to feel completely surrendered before beginning, so that there is no *nen* at work in your own heart-mind.

3. Place one hand at the back of the head, near the point at which the spine connects to the client's skull.

4. Place your other hand over the client's forehead and draw the *sei heki* symbol.* Allow Reiki to flow between your hands and visualize the symbol flowing between your hands as well. Proceed to step 5 when you begin to feel the energy saturating the area.

5. Repeat the affirmation three times. Do so out loud if possible. Your client can repeat the affirmation out loud or silently.

6. Remove your hand from your client's forehead. Continue to give Reiki to the base of the skull for approximately fifteen minutes. (Optionally, both hands may be placed on the back of the client's head, stacked one on top of the other at this point.) Try to recite the affirmation to yourself if your mind begins to wander.

7. Afterward, resume *gasshō* and bow to your client. Allow him or her to rest for a few moments before speaking or otherwise interacting. You can take this time to use *kenyoku hō* to disconnect from the client's energy altogether.

❂ *Sei Heki Chiryō Hō* 性癖治療法

The original method of employing the harmony symbol probably resembles the technique used in Jikiden Reiki and other Japanese lineages. It is a simple yet powerful method of effecting change at the psychological level. Although the technique below is similar to the way it's practiced in Jikiden, in order to respect the integrity of the lineage and teachings you will need to enroll in an

---

*I have found several variations in the exact procedures used in this technique. Although the steps are all very similar, the sequence differs from one tradition to the next. The *shirushi* may be drawn either at the back of the skull or at the forehead; experiment and find whichever sequence is best for your practice. I find it much easier to draw the *sei heki* on the forehead during self-treatment. Conversely, some versions (like that found in Petter's *This Is Reiki*) use no symbols at all.

okuden-level course with the Jikiden Reiki Kenkyukai to learn the technique precisely as Hayashi-sensei taught it.

Sei heki means "bad habit," and thus *sei heki chiryō hō* is the "method for bad habit treatment." It combines the power of the second *shirushi* with a command reaching into the subconscious. The original text recited by Hayashi is considered to have strong *kotodama.* The translation used below is found in *The Big Book of Reiki Symbols* by Walter Lübeck and Mark Hosak.[6]

The client should supply the issue or condition to be resolved. Rather than trying to place a positive spin on it, he or she should state it as simply and fundamentally as possible. By giving the client time to really sort out his or her way to the core concern, it may be revealed that the deepest layer of the issue is not as simple as feeling weak, having anxiety, or not having money.

The *sei heki chiryō* should be given for at least half an hour if possible. It's always better to begin with a hands-on treatment on the physical level first, given that the hands-on application of Reiki builds a rapport between practitioner and recipient. If your mind wanders, rein it in by reciting the *gokai* silently. Many clients experience a release, such as shedding of tears, during this treatment, so try to remain as detached as possible.

The real goal in both *sei heki chiryō* and *nentatsu hō* is the healing of the *kokoro.* Reiki helps polish the heart so that it is able to reflect the truth of who your client really is; their inner light will become increasingly visible whenever the second symbol is intentionally applied. As the harmony symbol works its way through the mind and heart together, it heals the rift between them and imparts a deep-seated peace and awareness of the infinite light within.

On a practical side, *sei heki chiryō* is very effective in cases of compulsion, addiction, negative self-image, bad habits, anxiety, depression, fears and phobias, relationship difficulties, and virtually any other condition that has a psychological origin. Yamaguchi Tadao (the son of Chiyoko Yamaguchi and the cofounder with her of Jikiden Reiki) even describes using this method successfully to command the consciousness of cells within the muscle, bone, and other tissues to correct physical conditions.[7]

1. Place the hands in *gasshō* and bow to your client.
2. With one hand, draw the *sei heki* symbol over the client's crown.[8]

3. Recite the following: "Human Being, Crown of Creation, stop _____ and return to your natural, normal state."⁹ (Fill in the blank space with the issue to be resolved.)

4. Hold your hand in place above the crown of your client's head for the duration of the treatment. Switch hands if your arm tires. You may feel *byōsen*-like sensations, but please do not use the power symbol to disrupt them.

5. When you are finished, resume *gasshō* and bow once more. You may follow up with *kenyoku hō.*

❈ *Enkaku Chiryō Hō* 遠隔治療法

The method for distance healing that originates from Japan is called *enkaku chiryō hō,* which translates to "remote treatment method" in English. The Japanese technique is ideologically similar to methods in Western branches of Reiki; I love that it makes use of the practitioner's body as the surrogate. Practicing in this way helps establish a more profound connection between client and practitioner and cultivates greater compassion and empathy.

One of the other benefits of *enkaku chiryō* is that it can be easier to sense *byōsen* when one's hands are on a living thing, as compared to the previously described methods of distance healing. There is a small chance that you may sense some of your own *byōsen,* so practice often until the difference may be discerned. Regular self-treatment will also reduce the interference of your *byōsen* with that of your clients.

As described in chapter 17 about the *HSZSN* symbol, gather as much information about the client as possible; a photograph makes the connection much easier. The practitioner will "project the image of the receiver onto a part of your own body."¹⁰ This could be a thigh, a finger, or the back of the arm, for instance. Imagine that the recipient is facing whichever way will make it easier for treatment, as if he or she were stretched out on your leg instead of a massage table.

Remember that the *HSZSN* is a *jumon,* and its power comes from being spoken. If you cannot speak the mantra out loud, you can silently affirm it to yourself as you draw the symbol. Use it to treat friends, family, and clients who live far away, or treat yourself in locations that are hard to reach, like your back or the kidneys. It can also be combined with other techniques such as *byōsen reikan hō* (scanning for *byōsen*), *reiji hō* (finding guidance through Reiki), *sei heki chiryō hō* (mental-emotional healing), or any of the Western innovations such as Aura Sweeping or the Chakra Tune-Up.

1. Start in *gasshō* and connect to Reiki.
2. Choose the part of your body that is serving as the surrogate, such as your leg or palm. Picture your client there, with his or her head at your knee and his or her feet by your hip.
3. Draw the *HSZSN* atop the image of your client. Recite its mantra three times.
4. Treat whichever target areas you would normally treat in person. Use the *choku rei* to empower or focus on specific areas or whenever you encounter *byōsen*. Additional techniques may also be practiced.
5. When you are finished, follow your standard closing procedures if time permits, just as you would if you were treating the client in person.

❂ *Enkaku Byōsen Reikan Hō* 遠隔病腺靈感法

As is true of the previous technique, *enkaku byōsen reikan hō* offers *okuden* practitioners the opportunity to work remotely in order to provide care for clients. The name of this technique is a combination of two others; it's roughly translated as "remote *byōsen* scanning method." Practitioners can take advantage of the connection *jumon* to intuitively scan a client's energy field or body for areas of disharmony.

In cases of distance healing, *enkaku byōsen reikan hō* is an obvious means for Reiki practitioners to familiarize themselves with their clients' state of being. However, this diagnostic procedure is also a welcome tool for in-person treatments and self-healing. When seeking *byōsen* through conventional hands-on means, the rhythmic processes of the physical body can muddy one's perceptions, at times making it difficult to discern *byōsen* from biological activity. On oneself it's especially difficult to clearly delineate these processes from their energetic counterparts. This is the perfect opportunity to use the distance method instead.

Since *enkaku* methods utilize the thigh, where there is little chance of finding your own *byōsen,* it's virtually impossible to get mixed messages through *enkaku byōsen reikan.* When working on yourself or a client, scanning remotely—even though you have hands-on access—ensures accuracy and speed in searching for areas of disharmony. After locating *byōsen,* switch to hands-on treatment for the remainder of the session; you will more than likely feel the *byōsen* clearly in the place(s) determined by remote scanning.

1. Start in *gasshō* and connect to Reiki.
2. Choose the part of your body serving as the surrogate, such as your leg. Picture your client there, with his or her head at your knee and his or her feet by your hip.
3. Draw the *HSZSN* atop the image of your client. Recite its mantra three times.
4. Place your hands, with palms still together, at your brow. Two variations exist: one with the fingertips pointed at the point between your eyebrows, and a second with the thumbs resting there instead.
5. Offer a prayer or statement of intent such as "I ask that the consciousness of Reiki guide my hands on behalf of my client."
6. Use the hand with which you have drawn the connection *jumon* to sweep slowly through your client's energy field, beginning approximately one foot above the head. Move your hand slowly and deliberately, noting any changes in the quality of the flow of Reiki. Wherever you feel *byōsen,* make a mental note.
7. Treat the area that has the highest intensity of *byōsen* first.

❈ *Shashin Chiryō Hō* 写真治療法

A variation on *ekaku chiryō, shashin chiryō* means "photograph treatment," and it was a favorite of Usui-sensei himself. He apparently used distance healing with great frequency, especially after the Great Kanto Earthquake.[11] Similar techniques are still used today in Japan, and the following method is inspired by the version taught by Koyama Kimiko, former president of the Usui Reiki Ryōhō Gakkai.[12]

In Usui-sensei's lifetime, photographs were relatively uncommon in most Japanese households—only the wealthiest individuals could afford them. As a result, Usui offered other means of utilizing the *jumon* for distance healing. Students who lived contemporaneously with Usui Mikao were said to have made quick drawings of clients, labeled with their names, in order to use *shashin chiryō hō* without access to photos. Reiki practitioners today frequently engage in similar methods when practicing long-distance healing.

Using a photograph enables the practitioner to touch painful or otherwise inappropriate parts of the body as necessary, unlike a treatment offered in person. Rather than simply using the photograph to make a connection, the photo is treated as if it were the client; remember that these distance healing methods merely use props as a tool for focusing the mind.

1. Begin as before, in *gasshō,* and connect to Reiki.
2. Hold the photograph or place it on a flat surface in front of you. Draw the *jumon* in the air over the photo and recite its mantra.
3. Place your hands on the photo for treatment. You can cover the entire person with the whole hand or use the fingertips of the first and/or second finger to localize the treatment to the parts of the client's body relevant to the condition. As before, other methods or *shirushi* may be employed, just as would be done in a face-to-face treatment.

The following chapter will walk you through best practices that have evolved out of Western Reiki lineages, including programming crystals with the symbols and a discussion of how Reiki can be stored for future use. It will also detail how Reiki can help with sleep and offer up some meditations that can be done in conjunction with the symbols.

19

ADDITIONAL *OKUDEN* TOOLS AND TECHNIQUES

THE METHODS OUTLINED in this chapter are extended techniques in the Reiki milieu. Most have been developed as additional tools and practices by practitioners of Western Reiki lineages; their present forms date to the death of Hawayo Takata in 1980. I've collected these exercises from many sources and lineages; the versions described below are distilled from my experience. Although most of them are not extant in *dento Reiki* or traditional Western Reiki, each of these has gained popularity in many Reiki communities worldwide.

✦ Programming Crystals and Gemstones with the Symbols

This method is inspired by Usui Mikao's use of quartz crystals to provide Reiki to clients who lived too far away to take the training themselves. Clear quartz is the premier choice, but other gemstones and minerals may be selected according to particular need as the scenario dictates. Reiki-charged crystals make wonderful gifts and can also be placed in strategic locations for healing the Earth and all who come near them. You can choose to use a single *shirushi* or *jumon,* or you can use them all at once. I usually follow up any single use or combination of *sei heki* and *HSZSN* with the focus symbol to amplify and empower the symbols. The crystals can then be used for Reiki-charged crystal grids, placed on a person for healing, or carried with you for extra support.

1. Cleanse the crystal beforehand; try using *jaki kiri jōka hō.*

2. Hold the crystal between your palms as you hold your hands in *gasshō* and connect to Reiki. Focus on your intention to charge the crystal.

3. Place the crystal in the open palm of your nondominant hand. Draw the *shirushi* or *jumon* you've chosen vertically over the crystal with the other hand, repeating its mantra three times.

4. With your dominant hand, sweep the symbol down toward the crystal and tap it three times.

5. When all of the selected symbols have been drawn and placed in the crystal, hold it between your hands in *gasshō* and reflect on your intention.

6. If possible, repeat once each week or whenever the crystal's charge appears to wane.

❖ The Reiki Box

Reiki is such a versatile tool that it can be applied using many different methods. This extended technique makes use of this versatility and allows you to exercise your creativity. Once you've created a Reiki box, your goals, Reiki requests, and affirmations may be placed inside it in order to dose them with good vibes around the clock. After Reiki boxes became popular, crafters and artisans began to design and sell elaborately adorned versions; making your own can be extremely satisfying.

Using your Reiki box allows you to send gentle and continuous Reiki to all the people you encounter who make special requests for healing. You can also place your intentions and manifestation goals therein as a means of enhancing your process. Update the contents frequently so that you can celebrate all of your successes and streamline where the energy is flowing. I like to keep Reiki-infused crystals in my Reiki box as well.

1. Make, decorate, or purchase a box or container. Consider drawing the kanji for Reiki (靈氣), writing the Five Principles, adding words, affirmations, or symbols of healing, and even adding crystals and gemstones. If you'd like to include the *jumon* and *shirushi,* consider placing them inside the box where they will remain out of sight.

2. Consecrate and empower your box. You can light some incense or sage and waft the smoke over it, sprinkle it with blessed (and Reiki-charged) water or salt, or simply pray over it. Place your hands on or over the box and recite the Five Principles.

3. Draw the three Reiki symbols in the air over the box and recite their mantras three times.

4. Affirm or state your intention for the Reiki box: that it will be a sacred vessel for magnifying, directing, and focusing Reiki on the intentions, goals, and recipients identified within it.

5. Add your Reiki requests. You can place notes, photos, written affirmations and intentions, or other reminders of where the Reiki will go. Add crystals, stones, feathers, shells, or other tokens of healing to your box as you feel inspired to do so.

6. Each day or whenever you have time, place your hands over the box and give it Reiki in order to focus healing on its contents.

7. Once a week or so, empty the box and remove the papers that pertain to what has come to fruition. Return the rest of the works in progress to the vessel and re-empower the box with the three symbols.

❖ Your Reiki Bank Account

Many of us have found ourselves in situations that could have been made easier with a little extra Reiki. It's impossible to plan for every circumstance and send Reiki in advance accordingly. However, there is a technique that can be used to help in these instances. I ran across a similar technique to the one outlined below in a Reiki book published in India some years ago. I loved the idea of sending Reiki to a universal "bank account" to be saved for when an extra boost is needed. Deposits and withdrawals can be made at any time.

There is no literal location, etheric or physical, that allows one to store Reiki or "earn interest" on it. However, the universe holds miracles for us in divine trust whenever we are not ready to receive or exercise them. Using the same law, we can prepare for future emergencies by sending Reiki to be held in a similar fashion. The key here is to clearly visualize or focus on your intent because the "moving force of this concept is its intention. What you are basically doing is collecting your intention."[1]

Ideally, you can practice this technique each day or whenever there isn't another pressing need to focus Reiki in the present moment, such as when you are generally healthy. Regular "deposits" ensure that you will have additional support waiting when you encounter a crisis or another situation that calls for an enhanced need for Reiki. Although the Reiki "bank account" may be practiced without the symbols, it is much more effective after the *okuden* training, at which point you can empower your intention with the *shirushi* and *jumon.*

1. Place your hands in *gasshō* and connect to Reiki.
2. Imagine a crystal box or cube floating ahead of you; this is your Reiki bank. Draw the *HSZSN* and beam Reiki from your hands into the container.
3. Allow Reiki to flow into the box for as long as you like; this vessel has no limit to the amount of energy it can hold. When you are done, draw the *choku rei* to seal the box and anchor the process.
4. Whenever you find yourself in a position in which you need an additional Reiki boost, draw or visualize the *HSZSN* in order to connect to your Reiki bank. Ask that the stored energy flow through you in addition to your normal flow of energy.
5. Place your hands (or breath, eyes, and intention) as needed.
6. Afterward, seal the box again using the *choku rei.* Repeat filling and using the energy in the crystalline box as often as you need to.

❖ Better Sleep with the Reiki Symbols

If getting a full night's rest is an elusive goal, Reiki can support relaxation and deeper sleep. When you use the first two *shirushi* in combination to clear the space and calm the mind, your bedroom becomes a safe haven for slumber. Follow up with some hands-on healing in bed until you drift away to dreamland.

1. Stand or sit in your bedroom in *gasshō* and recite the *gokai* in whichever form you feel most connected to.
2. Draw the *choku rei* on your hands and tap your palms together three times.
3. Draw the *choku rei* on the walls, ceiling, and floor of your bedroom.
4. Draw the *sei heki* over the bed.
5. Climb into bed and offer yourself hands-on Reiki as you fall asleep.

❖ Symbol Meditation

The Reiki symbols are powerful catalysts for healing and spiritual development. They can be harnessed in hands-on healing as well as in your personal meditation. The following technique is a simple method to help you become intimately familiar with the energetic signature of each of the *shirushi* and *jumon*. You may choose to visualize the symbol or draw it on paper and gaze upon it during meditation.

As you get to know the symbols for healing, it helps if you can deepen your bond with them. There are many ways to do this, the primary one being to practice them at every opportunity. Draw them in the air and pull them into your energy field. Use them for self-healing practice. Try them out with friends. Most importantly, you can use them in meditation. Doing so will bring you insight into their deeper meanings and empower you to integrate their effects into your energy field. Practice the following, one symbol at a time, until you have worked with each of them.

1. Decide whether you will draw or merely imagine the symbol. Find a quiet place and dim the lighting.
2. Place your hands in *gassho* and quiet your mind. Set your intention to connect to the chosen *shirushi* or *jumon*.
3. Using your dominant hand, draw the symbol in the air in front of you. Recite its mantra three times, out loud if possible.
4. Connect to the symbol by projecting it onto your mental screen or by gazing at it for the duration of your meditation.
5. When you are finished, draw the symbol in the air and repeat its mantra three times.
6. Place your hands in *gassho* and give thanks.

At this point you have many tools in your Reiki toolbox. No doubt they will enhance your own self-healing by empowering your practice. The next section of the book, its conclusion, will briefly summarize what we have learned about Reiki.

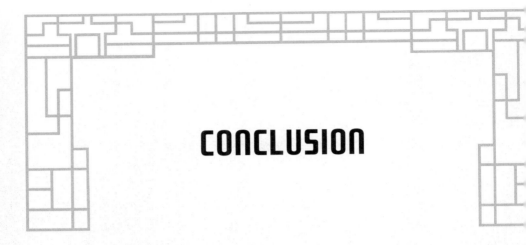

CONCLUSION

REIKI IS A POPULAR TOOL because of its efficacy and simplicity. However, after working through the theory and practice in this volume, you will see that Reiki Ryōhō is much more than just a method of healing with your hands. Reiki offers tools to transform your life from the inside out, and it will grow with you forevermore. Some of the key takeaways about Reiki can be summarized as thus:

- Reiki is natural, effective, universal, intelligent, and easy.
- Reiki is innately spiritual.
- Reiki propels both physical and mental-emotional healing.
- Reiki is an exercise in surrender.
- Practice makes perfect.

REIKI IS . . .

It's not always easy to describe Reiki to others, especially given the context of the energy of Reiki versus the practice of Usui Reiki Ryōhō. The characters for *rei* and *ki* in Japanese have complex layers of meaning, and the English language lacks comparable depth. Reiki is a natural force or energy inherent in all forms. Everything with life has Reiki; it is within each of us from the moment we're born.

Reiki is an effective tool in part because of its universality, but also because of its inherent intelligence. This intelligent force meets us where we are the most ready to be healed. Learning Reiki is simple—all we need are training and the initiations in order to practice it for life.

Reiki Ryōhō is the art of cultivating a relationship with the Reiki present in us all. As practitioners we are conduits rather than healers. The recipient of Reiki healing is actually the one doing all of the healing, for Reiki provides the energy necessary to return to homeostasis. Our only job is to show up, compassionately and fully present.

THE SPIRITUALITY OF REIKI

Usui Mikao did not climb Mount Kurama in order to obtain a miraculous healing ability. Rather, he made his journey and began a fast in order to achieve awakening so that he could achieve *anshin ritsumei*. After his enlightenment experience in which he was struck by *dai Reiki* (great Reiki), he *accidentally* discovered that he had received the ability to heal.

The goal of Reiki Ryōhō is personal development, ultimately aimed at reaching *anshin ritsumei*. This is a state of complete peace of mind, totally undisturbed by worry, anger, fear—or anything else. From this position, we are able to accomplish the divine mission for which our life is destined. Usui's purpose was to heal, and that's how Reiki was born.

Usui-sensei named his system Shin Shin Kaizen Usui Reiki Ryōhō: the Usui Reiki Healing Method for Improving the Heart-Mind and Body. Its primary emphasis is on inner healing. Physical wellness is a symptom of a balanced heart-mind, and so we engage in physical healing to clear away whatever is inhibiting our growth. Reiki provides for us on all levels.

PRACTICE, PRACTICE, PRACTICE . . .

One of the most unique aspects of Reiki is that we need only the initiation to be able to tap into the vast wellspring of Reiki energy for healing. However, the application of Reiki Ryōhō is like any other skill, and it must be refined through practice. Usui gave us the road map for both the inner and outer components of Reiki. This is why the *gokai* and the Japanese Reiki Techniques are such valuable stepping-stones along the way to mastering it.

If you seek deeper healing, the most important factor is your practice. Give yourself Reiki daily. Recite the precepts and endeavor to live by them. Offer Reiki to your loved ones as much as you can. Share it with your pets and charge your food and water with Reiki. Reiki is the best teacher, and you can only engage with this teacher by spending time with it.

Before students in Japan advance to *shinpiden,* or the third degree, they often spend years at each of the first two levels of Reiki. Although such a long time may not be entirely necessary, we can learn from their example by dedicating ourselves to our work. This is the true meaning of the fourth precept!

GROWING YOUR PRACTICE

When you are comfortable with the basic levels of Reiki, it is natural to want to share it with the world. Practitioners can harness the efficacy of Reiki as a professional practice in addition to a personal one. Network with other healers and bodyworkers and learn from the trends in your community. If you'd like to deepen your practice as well as create a thriving profession of Reiki, you can work toward building a clientele.

Many people who learn Reiki also love to share with others in their local Reiki community. Look for local Reiki circles, Reiki shares, and other events. Some teachers offer special workshops and seminars: classes in the Japanese Reiki Techniques, talks about the *gokai,* and/or special methods and applications, such as Reiki for children or animals. By networking with your local Reiki community you may find many ways to support one another and continue to grow.

Giving back is a drive that many of us have in the Reiki world. Today many hospitals, hospices, and shelters offer Reiki services. Practitioners of its many branches also band together to offer Reiki to animals, veterans, seniors, and patients coping with critical illness. When we really commit to our practice, there are many opportunities to grow and give back.

LET REIKI TEACH YOU

Hawayo Takata's most famous injunction to her students was, "Let Reiki teach you." Only by giving our whole hearts (or *kokoro*) to our Reiki practice can we learn authentically. Reiki Ryōhō is a healing system that focuses on the inner and spiritual aspects of our being first; it confers all the tools necessary to polish the heart so that it will reflect the great shining light of the soul's true nature.

Reiki asks us to have faith and to surrender. We learn to trust that Reiki works, mostly through the evidence that we accrue along the way. This spiritual rain of miracles is never ending; Reiki cannot be exhausted or depleted. When we put our faith in the higher powers of the universe, we are always taken care of.

When you feel drawn to learn the third degree, prepare yourself by living the Reiki lifestyle. Instead of merely repeating the Five Principles, act them out each day. Instead of thinking about how great Reiki is, demonstrate the depth and beauty of its benefits through your practice. Let it be your truest friend and most trusted teacher.

Shinpiden means "mystery teachings"; the third degree introduces us to the most profound mysteries of the Usui System of Natural Healing. However, after undergoing *shoden* and *okuden,* you already have those seeds planted within you. Tend to them through daily practice of Reiki, and they will soon blossom!

APPENDIX A

SUBTLE ANATOMY

A DISCUSSION OF REIKI would not be complete without specific attention paid to the body's subtle anatomy, for Reiki works with all aspects of the subtle anatomy to do its healing work. Components of subtle anatomy include the chakras and the different energy bodies that surround the physical body. The subtle anatomy is also made up of the *tanden,* the three energy centers of the body. We will delve a bit more deeply into these topics below. Though traditional Reiki does not include teachings about the aura or chakras, many students find this information helpful for enhancing their practice.

THE AURA

The aura is the electromagnetic field that surrounds and penetrates the physical body. The aura itself is shaped like a torus; the physical body stands in the center of the opening within it.

Various different layers of the human energy field have their own function, such as the etheric body, mental body, emotional body, and causal body. It is possible to sense *byōsen* in the energy bodies of the aura.

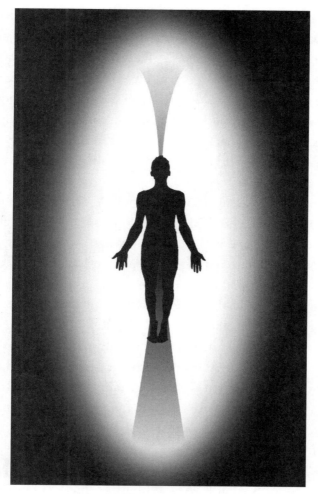

The aura reflects one's emotional, spiritual, mental, and physical condition. Each person's aura is unique.

THE CHAKRA SYSTEM

The chakra system was only introduced to Reiki after the year 1980, when Hawayo Takata passed away. Most updates to Usui Shiki Ryōhō that employed the chakras are likely to have occurred during the 1990s, when Reiki underwent rapid change due to globalization. Even though Usui never touched upon the subject of the chakras, they're a viable and easily understood aspect of our subtle anatomy. The word *chakra* (which is pronounced with a hard *ch* as in *cheer*) is derived from the Sanskrit *cakram,* meaning "wheel." The chakras are centers of vital energy shaped more or less like spinning wheels, or spiraling vortices, that are accessible from both the front and the back of the body.

Quick and effective Reiki treatments can consist of treating each of the chakras. Although this is not a part of *dento Reiki,* many teachers and students make use of the chakra system today. Brief descriptions of each of the chakras follow.

The root chakra lies at the base of the spine, though it is sometimes visualized at the perineum. Most people picture the root chakra as being red. It is associated with survival, strength, and being grounded. The root chakra is connected to abundance, motivation, and kundalini. Its domain in the physical body includes any aspect related to survival, strength, and movement: the bones, muscles, circulatory system, metabolism, and reproductive organs.

The sacral chakra is located approximately one and one-half to two inches below the navel. Associated with the color orange, the second chakra represents connection, sexuality, vitality, passion, creativity, and fertility. It rules the reproductive organs, kidneys, and bladder and connects us to our emotions on a primal level.

The third chakra is located at the solar plexus, which is centered just below the sternum. This yellow energy center is connected to personal power, will, manifestation, intellect, and self-esteem. In the physical body the solar plexus relates to the organs of the digestive system, the adrenal glands, and the diaphragm. It also vitalizes the eliminatory functions of the body, including those of the urinary tract, liver, lungs, and skin.

The fourth chakra, or heart center, is in the center of the chest. Many practitioners use green and/or pink to represent the heart chakra. Its energetic rulership includes the emotions, love, higher-level relationships, balance, and compassion. Physiologically, this energy center is tied to the heart and circulatory system, immune system, respiratory system, and our overall sense of well-being. It is the cen-

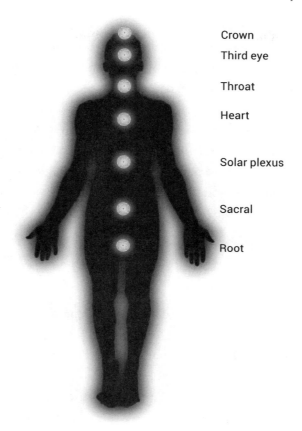

Crown
Third eye
Throat
Heart
Solar plexus
Sacral
Root

The seven chakras of the human body

ter of our energy field and is the primary sensory organ of the subtle anatomy.

The next chakra is located at the throat and is envisioned as blue. The throat center relates to communication, self-expression, truth, and putting our mental energy into form. On the physical level, it relates to the mouth, throat, nervous system and sensory organs, and thyroid glands.

The sixth chakra is usually associated with the color indigo and is located between and slightly above the eyebrows. Known as the third-eye chakra, this energy center represents the higher function of the mind, dreaming, intuition, purpose, and understanding. The third eye is related to the eyes, sinuses, brain (especially the pineal gland), and sensory organs of the head. It helps mediate between the higher planes and the material plane by providing insights into the underlying spiritual forms of our experiences in the everyday world.

The seventh chakra is at the crown of the skull. The crown center is usually pictured as violet or white; it's representative of our divine connection. It rules the brain, nervous system, pituitary gland, and subtle anatomy. The crown center is the channel through which Reiki enters the practitioner's system. This chakra represents our ability to surrender, access higher consciousness, and be a vessel for the Divine to work through us.

THE THREE *TANDEN*

The three *tanden* are fields or centers of energy that are recognized in Taoism and Buddhism. Originating in China, the word *tanden* is composed of characters that mean "red" or "crimson" (丹) and "field" or "rice paddy" (田). The term *red field* may poetically refer to the location (field) where the elixir of life or vital energy (red) is stored. Called *dantian* in Chinese, these energy centers are utilized in martial arts and spiritual practices with ties to Taoism. Although similar to the chakras, the major difference is that the *tanden* centers are viewed as storage centers in which qi or ki (氣) is transformed or converted into other forms. The concepts of the aura and chakras were absent from Usui's original teachings on Reiki Ryōho, but he did include information on the *tanden,* as is evidenced in a number of the Japanese Reiki Techniques.

Lower *Tanden: Shimotanden* 下丹田

The lower *tanden* is the home of our personal, vital power. It is also the most important of the *tanden* in the original Reiki teachings. Hawayo Takata often described the lower *tanden* as the battery or "big motor" of the body. Reiki flows down through our divine connection at the crown of the head and into the lower *tanden* before being channeled

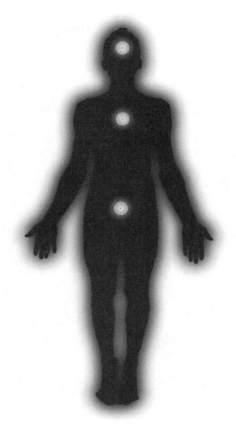

The three *tanden* are the upper, middle,
and lower energy centers, as highlighted here.

outward for healing. Breathing consciously into the *shimotanden* helps cultivate our ability to refine and expand the energy we store there.

The lower *tanden* is often referred to as the *hara* or abdomen in Japanese. It's visualized as the root of our energetic tree. The *hara* is the center of gravity, source of *prana* or vital energy, and the place from which our "gut" instincts spring.

Middle *Tanden*: Chūtanden 中丹田

The *chūtanden* dwells at the heart. Reiki moves upward from the lower *tanden* and passes through the heart before being directed through the eyes, hands, and breath for treatment. The middle *tanden* is considered the storage center for the energy of the spirit that flows with the breath. In Chinese, this is expressed as qi being converted to *shen*.

Upper *Tanden: Kamitanden* 上丹田

The upper *tanden* is less recognized for its functions in Reiki. In Taoism, the upper *tanden* is the site in which the spirit (*shen*) is converted to emptiness (*wu wei*). It resides at the brow or third eye.

PRONUNCIATION GUIDE

IN THE JAPANESE LANGUAGE, each vowel and consonant typically produces a single sound, with very few exceptions. Phonetically, Japanese is quite simple, with only a couple of sounds that may feel unfamiliar to a speaker of English.

VOWELS

- *a* sounds like *ah* as in f**a**ther.
- *e* is somewhere between the *eh* of **e**gg and *ay,* such as s**ay.**
- *i* produces the *ee* sound of the word b**ee**t.
- *o* is pronounced as *oh* and sounds like **vo**te or **co**at.
- *u* sounds like *oo* of f**oo**d.

CONSONANTS

- *b* sounds like the English equivalent, like **b**oy.
- *ch* is always like **ch**ange.
- *d* is identical to English, as in **d**og.
- *f* is sometimes a bit breathier than in English but otherwise sounds similar to **f**eel.
- *g* is always hard, as in **g**oal.
- *h* sounds like **h**ouse.

- *j* is hard, as in **j**ump.
- *k* is just as it is in English, such as **k**iss.
- *m* is the same also, such as **m**ud.
- *n* is the same as English at the beginning of a syllable, like **n**ame, but at the end of a syllable sometimes sounds like *m* (when it precedes *m, b,* or *p*) or *ng* (when it precedes *g* or *k*).
- *p* sounds like **p**at.
- *r* falls closer to the sound of an *l* or *d* in English, with a single flap against the roof of the mouth, just behind the teeth. Do not roll the Japanese *r*.
- *s* sounds like **s**imple.
- *t* makes the same sound in both languages, as in **t**ouch.
- *ts* is found at the start of the syllable in Japanese, although it sounds as it does in ha**ts**.
- *w* is usually pronounced as **w**ash, except in the particle *wo,* in which the *w* is silent.
- *y* sounds like **y**es, and it can also be used in diphthongs, explained below.
- *z* sounds just like **z**oo.

COMPOUNDS WITH Y

The Japanese syllables *ya, yu,* and *yo* can be combined with most consonants, such as in the words *ryōhō* and *byōsen.* These words should pronounce the *y* and the vowel following it in a single syllable. For example, *byōsen* is not pronounced as *bee yoh sen* or as *bye yoh sen.* The consonant preceding the *y* is pronounced with the *y* and the vowel immediately thereafter in one single syllable.

LONG VOWELS, SILENT VOWELS, AND PAUSES

In the Japanese language, vowel length is a matter of duration of sound. Long vowels are transliterated with a macron above them: *ā, ē, ī, ō, ū.*

They are held for twice the length of short vowels. Long vowels are also written as doubled letters, like *aa* or *uu,* and in combinations such as *ei* and *ou.*

Two vowels are sometimes silent in special cases. Except in some regional dialects, the letters *i* and *u* are not usually pronounced between unvoiced consonants like *k, t, s, f, ch,* and *ts.* For instance, the expression *kanshashite* is pronounced *kahn shah **shtay.***

Short pauses occur in Japanese pronunciation whenever a consonant is doubled, such as in the words *gasshō* and *gakkai.* Imagine a short, silent gap between the syllables.

PHONETIC PRONUNCIATION
OF THE *GOKAI*

招福の秘法   *Shō fuku no hihō* ("The secret method of inviting good fortune")
Shoh foo-koo no hee-hoh

萬病の靈薬   *manbyō no rei yaku* ("The spiritual medicine of all illness")
Mahn-byoh no ray yah-koo

今日丈けは   *Kyō dake wa* ("Today only")
Kyoh dah-kay wah

怒るな   *ikaru na* ("Anger not")
Ee-kah-roo nah

心配すな   *shinpaisu na* ("Worry not")
Sheem-pie-soo nah

感謝して   *kanshashite* ("Be grateful")
Kahn-shah shtay

業をはげめ   *gyō wo hageme* ("Be diligent in your work")
Gyoh-oh hah-gay-may

人に親切に   *hito ni shinsetsu ni* ("Be kind to people")
Hee-toh nee sheen-set-soo nee

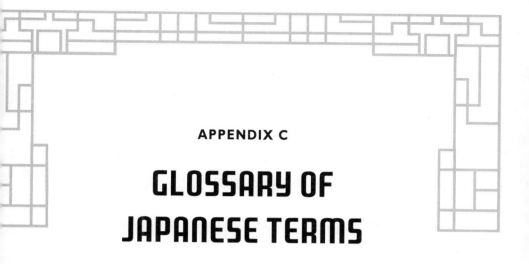

GLOSSARY OF JAPANESE TERMS

ame (雨): "Rain." This expression can be used figuratively to mean "spiritual rain" or "the infinite blessings that rain down from heaven." This character is a radical in the *rei* character of *Reiki* (靈 or 霊).

Amida Nyōrai (阿弥陀如来): Amida Nyōrai is the central figure in Jōdo Buddhism. Synonymous with Amitābha Tathagata and Amitāyus (both Sanskrit, meaning "infinite/boundless light" and "infinite/boundless life," respectively) and Āmítuófó (Chinese), Amida is known by many epithets, including Buddha of Boundless (or Infinite) Light, Buddha of Infinite Life, Buddha of Boundless Light and Consciousness, Buddha of Boundless Light and Life, and Buddha of Enlightenment. Amida is symbolized by the seed syllable *hrīḥ*. He is considered to be the creator or origin of Senju Kannon in some myths, such as those propagated in Japanese Reiki systems.

anshin ritsumei (安心立命): Different schools variously pronounce the characters as *anshin ritsumei, anjin ritsumei, anshin ryūmei, anjin ryūmei,* and *anshin ryūmyō.* This expression can be roughly translated as "inner peace," "spiritual peace," or "enlightenment." *Anshin ritsumei* is a state of deeply centered peace (*anshin,* 安心, or "secure heart-mind"), which enables one to accomplish one's life's purpose (立命, *ritsumei,* denotes "attaining your destiny"). This is the state of mind in which authentic spiritual revelation occurs, and sincere spiritual practice helps cultivate *anshin ritsumei*. Usui's real target was not physical or spiritual healing but a means of guiding practitioners to achieving *anshin ritsumei*.

atsui onnetsu (熱い温熱): Literally "intense heat"; the second level of *byōsen*.

bonji (梵字): "Buddhist character." This is the Japanese term for the *siddham* script of the Sanskrit language. *Bonji* are common throughout Japan in Buddhist shrines and cemeteries, and Japan remains one of the most prolific users of the *siddham* script. These characters often represent Buddhas and bodhisattvas; they can be likened to monosyllabic mantras and work as visual representations of these figures. The second *shirushi* is derived from the *bonji* of Amida Nyōrai and Senju Kannon, *hrīḥ* (pronounced *kiriiku* in Japanese).

byōgen (病元): "The origin of disease." This refers to the home of the underlying pattern of energy, pathogen, injury, or imbalance that has caused illness. Often this will be the place where the greatest *byōsen* can be felt, although it is not always proximal to the symptoms. Treating the origin of a concern rather than only its symptoms will lead to faster and more efficient recovery and may prevent the same condition from recurring. The *byōgen* can often be found in the subtle bodies of clients rather than in the physical.

byōsen (病腺): Literally "sick lump." *Byōsen* is an original word coined by Reiki founder Usui Mikao that refers to the different sensations that occur as Reiki flows through the practitioner's hands, especially when an area of injury or illness is being treated. In addition to the sensations themselves, the word *byōsen* also means the areas where toxins, both physical and energetic, have accumulated in the body.

byōsen reikan hō (病腺靈感法): Literally "method for spiritually sensing *byōsen*." This is a technique for scanning the person being treated in order to sense the most strategic places to treat.

chiryō (治療): "Therapy" or "treatment." This is the third of the Three Pillars of the Usui Reiki Ryōhō Gakkai. It refers to both simple hands-on healing as well as a number of other *gihō* or techniques that are aimed at healing and are taught in Reiki. Examples include *heso chiryō, koki hō,* and *tanden chiryō.*

choku rei (直靈): Literally "direct spirit/soul," *choku rei* is the name of the first *shirushi* as it's taught in Western branches of Reiki. The term *choku rei* is also found in several other spiritual traditions of Japan; it's believed to have Shinto origins. See also *naohi, naobi* and *ichirei shikon.*

dai Reiki (大靈氣): This term occurs on Usui Mikao's memorial stone at Saihōji in Tokyo. *Dai Reiki* literally means "great Reiki" or "big Reiki," and it refers to the experience of Usui's satori. The *dai Reiki* describes the great, cosmic Reiki of the universe that Usui experienced when he received his spontaneous transmission of light that awakened his latent ability to heal and brought Usui into a state of *anshin ritsumei.*

dai shihan (大師範): "Senior instructor," a title adopted by some Japanese Reiki organizations to indicate a teacher who is permitted to initiate and instruct other teachers. There is some debate about which of Usui's *shinpiden* students were considered *dai shihan,* for the only photos of the group label these individuals as *reijusha,* or "initiators." The title *dai shihan* is used today in the Jikiden Reiki Kenkyukai as well as in the Usui Reiki Ryōhō Gakkai.

denju (傳授 or 伝授): Comprised of the symbols for "transmission" and "to grant, give, or confer," *denju* means "initiation." More broadly it can imply a general transmission or instruction, or teaching, such as the Reiki seminar in its entirety. While it appears that *denju* was not synonymous with *reiju* in Reiki, the healing system called Tenohira Ryōji taught by one of Usui Mikao's students, Eguchi Toshihiro, did in fact use this term to mean "initiation."

dento (傳統 or 伝統): This Japanese term means "tradition," and it's sometimes used to mean traditional Reiki, as in *dento Reiki* (傳統靈氣). This generally refers to Reiki as it was taught by Usui Mikao and as preserved by the Usui Reiki Ryōhō Gakkai. Jikiden Reiki can also be considered a form of *dento Reiki,* as it is an unaltered form of practice.

dojo (道場): Although the term *dojo* is typically used for martial arts settings, it can also be applied to spiritual disciplines. The kanji comprising *dojo* (traditionally transliterated as *dōjō*) translate as "way" and "hall," thus making it the "hall in which the way is studied." The *do* (道) character is the *tao* of *Taoism,* and it can refer to more than a literal path or way. Usui and Hayashi both had their own dojos.

enkaku byōsen reikan hō (遠隔病腺靈感法): Meaning "remote method for spiritually sensing *byōsen,*" this technique allows second degree practitioners to seek *byōsen* when treating clients long distance.

enkaku chiryō hō (遠隔治療法): This is a term for the distance healing method, translated literally as "remote treatment method." Various styles of long-distance healing are taught in the second degree, and they require the use of the third "symbol" or *jumon,* called *hon sha ze shō nen.*

gainen (概念): This term, translating as "concept, idea, or notion," is often erroneously used in place of *gokai* in Reiki circles. It was introduced by Reiki revisionist Dave King in his system called Usui Dō (臼井道), an attempt to re-create the early teachings of Usui Mikao as they existed prior to the formation of Usui Reiki Ryōhō. The Usui Dō teachings are based on spurious claims lacking verifiable sources.

gakkai (合会): Simply meaning "association," "academic meeting," or "organization," *gakkai* is used as an abbreviation for Usui Reiki Ryōhō Gakkai, the organization founded by Usui in April 1922.

gasshō (合掌): This word consists of symbols meaning "unite" and "palm." *Gasshō* is a mudra formed by bringing the hands together in front of the chest, similar to the prayer position. *Gasshō* is used to unify the heart-mind prior to the traditional Japanese techniques as well as in the meditations taught by Usui-sensei. In Asia, *gasshō* may be used as a separate meditation (*gasshō meiso*), as a greeting, for showing thanks, as an apology, or to indicate reverence.

gedoku hō (解毒法): "Method for detoxification." This is a Japanese Reiki Technique that treats the *tanden* of the client as a means of promoting the body's natural detoxification processes. See also *tanden chiryō.*

gihō (技法): Meaning simply "technique," *gihō* is a term applied to any of the meditative or healing-oriented developmental tools taught in traditional Reiki in Japan, also called *dento Reiki*.

gokai (五戒): This word literally means "five admonitions." It's the Japanese term for the Five Principles (or precepts) handed down by Usui Mikao. The *gokai* are the framework of the Reiki system. Some Reiki scholars choose the term *gainen*, meaning "concept," "idea," or "notion" instead, despite a lack of historical precedent. In Japan, the terms *kyōgi* and *ikun* have also been used to describe, though not necessarily to replace, the term *gokai*.

gokai sansho (五戒三唱): This phrase literally means "three recitations of *gokai*." Before *reiju*, treatment, or meditation, the Five Principles are recited three times. They may also be chanted in a similar fashion in the morning and evening, as recommended by Usui in *gakkai* president Ushida's calligraphic version of the *gokai*. *Sansho* is a traditionally Buddhist practice, although reciting the Reiki precepts in this fashion has been used by the Usui Reiki Ryōhō, Hayashi Reiki Kenkyukai, and Jikiden Reiki Kenkyukai. Nowadays, many Western practitioners and teachers have reinstated *gokai sansho* one way or another into modern Reiki practice.

gyōshi hō (凝視法): "Staring method" is the practice of administering Reiki treatment with the eyes.

hara (腹): *Hara* often translates to "abdomen" or "belly" in modern usage, although it more specifically refers to an energy center below the navel. The *hara* is the lower *tanden,* and it is more or less analogous to the second chakra. Japanese culture places special emphasis on the *hara;* it is viewed as the storehouse of Reiki in the body of practitioners.

hatsurei hō (發靈法): Although this term means "method for generating soul/spirit," it actually refers to a set of meditations and exercises that enhance the practice of Reiki Ryōhō by cultivating a clearer vessel through which Reiki flows and developing greater sensitivity to *byōsen*. *Hatsurei hō* indicate the innately spiritual nature of Reiki; they include *gasshō meiso, kenyoku hō, jōshin kokyū hō,* and *seishin tōitsu*.

Hayashi Reiki Kenkyukai (林靈氣研究会): This is the Reiki organization founded by Hayashi Chūjirō after he received encouragement from Usui himself. Hayashi focused on a more clinical approach to Reiki and was a prolific teacher, traveling far and wide throughout Japan and eventually teaching even in Hawaii. Thanks to Hayashi and his inspired if not unconventional decision to teach Hawayo Takata, Reiki has spread throughout the world. The Hayashi Reiki Kenkyukai ceased activity several years after Hayashi's passing.

heikin jōka (平均浄化): *Heikin jōka* means "average purification" or "balanced cleansing." This principle describes how *byōsen* is usually deposited and subsequently eliminated more or less symmetrically in the body.

heso chiryō (臍治療): This word literally means "navel treatment," which is a Japanese Reiki Technique used during hands-on healing to control excess heat or fire ki in the body.

hibiki (響き): The third degree of *byōsen* literally means "throbbing," "pulsing," "tremor," or "echo." *Hibiki* is sometimes used interchangeably with *byōsen* by practitioners of some lineages.

hō (法): *Hō* can variously mean "method," "law," "rule," "dharma," "principle," "model," or "system." It's used in a variety of expressions in systems of Japanese Reiki, such as *gihō, kenyoku hō,* and *koki hō,* and in the first line of the *gokai's* title: *shō fuku no hihō.* In these instances it usually simply denotes a method or technique.

hon sha ze shō nen (本者是正念): This is a *jumon* or formula used in distance healing. Taught in *okuden* (second degree), this written formula is part symbol and part mantra and enables practitioners to treat clients remotely. Refer to chapter 17 for a complete discussion.

ichirei shikon (一靈四魂): In Shinto, in some martial arts, and in other spiritual practices in Japan, the philosophy of *ichirei shikon* describes the spiritual makeup of human beings. Roughly translated as "one soul, four spirits" (or even "one spirit, four souls"), this phrase indicates that the human soul is made of four components, called the *kushitama* (奇魂), *aratama* (荒魂), *nigitama* (和魂), and *sakitama* (幸魂). Collectively, these four essential qualities comprise the *naohi/naobi* (直靈) or *reikon* (靈魂).

ikun (遺訓): This term is used by Hayashi to introduce the *gokai* in the scroll he brushed by hand. It can mean simply "legacy" but is also a term used to describe someone's dying wish.

itami (痛み): *Itami* is literally "pain," the fifth and most intense level of *byōsen* described by Hayashi-sensei.

jaki kiri jōka hō (邪氣切り浄化法): This is a cleansing method of using Reiki energy on inanimate objects. The name of this technique translates as "cleansing method that cuts through negative energy."

Jikiden Reiki Kenkyukai (直傳靈氣研究会): *Jikiden* translates as "by direct transmission" and *kenkyukai* means "institute" or "study group." This is a modern Reiki organization founded to preserve the teachings of Hayashi Chūjirō, as taught by the Yamaguchi family of Japan. Mrs. Yamaguchi Chiyoko learned Reiki from Hayashi-sensei in 1938, and the Jikiden Reiki Kenkyukai was started in 1999 to codify and promote traditional Hayashi-style Reiki.

Jōdo Shū (浄土宗): This branch of Buddhism, translated as "Pure Land School," is the variety to which Usui Mikao adhered. He attended elementary school at a Pure Land temple in rural Taniai, and his ashes are interred at a Jōdo cemetery in Tokyo. Established in 1175, it is the most widely practiced form of Buddhism in Japan and is characterized by a focus on Amida Nyōrai, also called Amitabha and Chenrezig.

jōshin kokyū hō (浄心呼吸法): This meditative practice constitutes part of the *hatsurei hō* techniques. It translates as "purification by breath method."

jumon (呪文): This word translates as "incantation" or "spell." *Jumon* refers to the formulaic composition of words, typically kanji, for a spiritual purpose. One of the three traditional Reiki symbols is in reality a *jumon*, rather than a *shirushi*. The power of a *jumon* in the system of Reiki lies in the spoken word. The symbols themselves are merely everyday characters or kanji; they produce an effect because of the strong *kotodama* that animates them.

kami (神): Often translated as "god" or "spirit," *kami* denotes the divine consciousness of a natural feature, force, creature, or idea. Similar to the devas of Vedic literature, kami are found throughout Creation. Although there are some kami that have anthropomorphic personifications, many are merely numinous forces of nature rather than discrete entities.

kanji (漢字): Han (Chinese) character/symbols. These are the Chinese characters adopted and modified by the Japanese as a writing system; they form one of several character sets used in Japanese orthography. Kanji have a rich history, stretching back millennia to ancient China, and as such, they often convey many layers of meaning.

kenyoku hō (乾浴法): This is a self-purification technique translated as "dry bathing." Usually taught in the first degree, this Japanese Reiki Technique is the first step of *hatsurei hō*.

ki (氣 or 気): *Ki* originally derives from the Chinese *chi* or *qi,* meaning "breath" or "vapor." Similar to the English word *spirit,* which comes from the Latin *spiritus,* meaning "breath" or "air," *ki* means "the breath of life that animates physical form." It's not simply metabolic energy; instead ki is the life force that our souls need for sustenance. Ki exercises are the foundation of qigong, called *kiko* in Japan. Ki is also harnessed in many martial arts, meditative pursuits, and healing traditions.

kiriiku (キリーク): The Japanese approximation of the *bonji* or seed syllable *hrīḥ. Kiriiku* sounds like *kleek* or *kreek,* given that Japanese pronunciation does not allow for a more accurate rendering of *hrīḥ.*

koki hō (呼氣法): Literally meaning "breathing method," this technique allows practitioners to treat clients by administering Reiki with the breath.

kokoro (心): *Kokoro* means both "heart" and "mind" in Japanese, thus expressing a unity between these two concepts that traditionally are separate in Western culture. *Kokoro* can also mean "the heart of" (a person, place, or thing) in a metaphorical way, just as in English. This character is also read *shin, jin,* and *gokoro* in Japanese.

kokyū hō (呼吸法): Translated as "breathing techniques," *kokyū hō* are a collection of meditations and exercises that make use of the breath, including *koki hō* and *seishin tōitsu.*

kotodama (言靈 or 言魂): This Japanese expression means "soul of the word." All words, syllables, and phonemes have an inherent power in Japanese thought. The basic principle of *kotodama* is that the spiritual power of these sounds can be used to influence reality. Thus, *jumon,* mantras, prayers, and affirmations each utilize the essence of *kotodama* when spoken.

Kurama Yama (鞍馬山): Mount Kurama is the site of Usui's enlightenment. Its name roughly translates as "horse saddle mountain," a reference to its shape.

kyōgi (教義): *Kyōgi* means "doctrine" or "principle." The *gokai* are called *kyōgi* in the *Reiki Ryōhō Hikkei,* the manual used by the *gakkai* in Japan.

meiso (瞑想): *Meiso* means "meditation." Derived from the Chinese 瞑 (*ming*), meaning "to close the eyes," and 想, meaning "idea, thought," 想 combines the radicals for "observe carefully" with *kokoro* (心), implying "to observe the heart-mind." Therefore, meditation is observing one's heart-mind with closed eyes. *Meiso* is used in *gasshō meiso,* one of the Three Pillars of traditional Reiki Ryōhō in Japan.

naohi, naobi (直靈): This is an alternate reading of the kanji for *choku rei,* as used in the spiritual traditions of Japan. *Naohi* refers to the soul of a human being as it is directly created by the kami. It is usually believed that the naohi is comprised of four component souls or spirits. See also *ichirei shikon* and *choku rei.*

nentatsu hō (念達法): "Method for reaching above thought/intention/desire." One of the two methods for mental-emotional healing employed in traditional Japanese-style Reiki, *nentatsu hō* is used to empower an affirmation or outcome for healing or a change in behavior. See also *sei heki chiryō.*

Nihon, Nippon (日本): These words are indigenous names for Japan and mean "land of the rising sun." They are compounds of 日, meaning "sun" (and by extension "day"), and 本, here meaning "origin."

Nihon no Reiki gihō (日本の技法): "Japanese Reiki Techniques." See also *gihō*.

nisei (二世): *Nisei* is a Japanese term used in North and South America to refer to the children of Japanese immigrants, literally meaning "second generation." Hawayo Takata was nisei.

okuden (奥傳 or 奥伝): *Okuden* is the original name for the second degree of Reiki in Japanese. *Oku* (奥) is "inner part," and *den* (傳) is "to transmit, convey." Thus, *okuden* means "the inner teachings of Reiki" and implies a direct transmission of the knowledge from teacher to student.

onnetsu (温熱): "Heat, warmth"; the first level of *byōsen*.

Oomoto Kyō (大本教): *Oomoto Kyō* is a "Japanese New Religion" or "new religious movement" (see entry below for *shinshūkyō*), founded in 1892 by Deguchi Nao. *Oomoto Kyō* means "Great Origin teachings." Since Oomoto was founded during Usui Mikao's lifetime and makes use of several terms extant in Reiki Ryōhō, many researchers have claimed that Usui and the founders of Oomoto may have known or learned from one another despite the lack of any concrete evidence to support their claims.

piri-piri kan (ピリピリ感): *Piri-piri kan* literally means "tingling sensation" and is the third level of *byōsen*.

rei (靈 or 霊): *Rei* is a kanji that denotes something inherently spiritual and esoteric. Its interpretations include "ghost," "soul," "spirit," "spiritual," "universal," "miraculous," "effective," "occult," "ancestral," and "intelligent." See chapter 1 for a complete discussion of the etymology and meaning of *rei*.

reiji hō (靈示法): One of the Three Pillars of Reiki in the *gakkai*, *reiji hō* means "method of indication by spirit." It is used to intuit the most effective place to treat a client with Reiki, given that it's used to locate *byōsen*.

reiju (靈授): The Japanese equivalent of the Western-style initiation or attunement in Reiki. *Reiju* means "spiritual offering" and provides the recipient with the *initial* (hence the term *initiation*) experience of their inner connection to Reiki and their true self. Japanese lineages that are preserved in the Usui Reiki Ryōhō Gakkai and in Jikiden Reiki uphold Usui-sensei's belief that students benefit from frequent *reiju*. In sharp contrast, most Western lineages purport that a single attunement is sufficient to practice Reiki.

Reiki (靈氣 or 霊気): "Spiritually guided life force" or "universal life force" are among the most common translations of this term, which has many meanings in modern and archaic Japanese. A more accurate translation might be "soul energy/life force" or "miraculous energy/life force." Please see chapter 1 for a complete discussion of these kanji. Nowadays, Reiki is often written in katakana (レイキ), the syllabary reserved mostly for foreign loanwards, to avoid the unpleasant connotations of the character *rei*.

Reiki Ryōhō (靈氣療法): Meaning "Reiki Healing Method," this expression today implies the system of Reiki, rather than merely the energy of Reiki. Before Usui-sensei's experience on Mount Kurama, other "spiritual energy healing methods" were in use in Japan, so he named his system Usui Reiki Ryōhō, or more formally Shin Shin Kaizen Usui Reiki Ryōhō, to set it apart from other healing modalities.

Reiki Ryōhō Hikkei (靈氣療法必携): This is a booklet given to members of the Usui Reiki Ryōhō Gakkai. The title of this document means "Reiki Healing Method Manual." The booklet consists of two main parts, the first of which is a question-and-answer style of explaining Reiki Ryōhō, while the second is a set of recommended hand placements to treat specific conditions. Translations have been made available in a number of Reiki books. This is one of the most important resources for understanding the Japanese perspective and roots of the Reiki tradition. Note that the "interview" portion of the text has been compiled and edited from earlier sources, which are currently unknown or unavailable.

Reiki Ryōhō no Shiori (靈氣療法のしおり): This "Reiki Ryōhō Guidebook" is a short book published by the Usui Reiki Ryōhō Gakkai in 1974. It includes a summary of Reiki history, theory, and practice.

ryōhō (療法): This word translates to "healing method." Reiki is one of many *ryōhō* in use today. Occasionally this word can also be translated as "cure."

satori (悟り): *Satori* means "enlightenment," "understanding," or "comprehension." It can be used to describe a personal awakening, such as Usui's episode on Mount Kurama. *Satori* is also arguably the goal of practicing Usui Reiki Ryōhō, as it reflects the attainment of *anshin ritsumei*.

sei heki (性癖): Literally "bad habit"; the modern connotation in Japan is more along the lines of "vice," "kink," or "perversion." This is used as the name of the second *shirushi* in Takata-derived lineages of Reiki. In Japanese Reiki Ryōhō this symbol is called *sei heki chiryō no shirushi*, or "symbol for treatment of bad habits." The *sei heki* is also known as the mental-emotional healing symbol and the harmony symbol.

sei heki chiryō (性癖治療法): The original prescribed use of the second *shirushi* is *sei heki chiryō*, or "bad habit treatment." It is used in the treatment of bad habits and mental-emotional conditions. See also *nentatsu hō*.

seishin tōitsu (精神統一): *Seishin tōitsu* is the final stage of *hatsurei hō* and literally means "spiritual unity" or "unification and purification of the spirit." It is a meditation traditionally taught in Japanese schools of Reiki.

seiza (正座): The Japanese style of sitting on the knees with the feet beneath you is called *seiza* or "correct sitting." Many of the Japanese Reiki Techniques are traditionally performed in *seiza*, and students also sit in *seiza* to receive *reiju* in Japan.

Senju Kannon (千手観音): Senju Kannon is the Japanese title for Avalokiteshvara or Guan Yin (Kuan Yin) with a thousand arms. Typically depicted somewhat androgynously, Senju Kannon holds a different implement in each hand, symbolically representing every remedy for suffering experienced by the human race. Senju Kannon is closely related to Amida Nyōrai (Amitabha Tathagata), the Buddha of Boundless Light. For this reason, they share the same Sanskrit seed syllable, which serves as the basis for the harmony symbol.

sensei (先生): This is a suffix applied to someone's name in order to indicate respect. As a title, it might indicate that the one being addressed is a teacher, instructor, doctor, or other professional of respectable status. Note that one never addresses oneself with this title (I would never call myself Pearson-sensei or Nicholas-sensei). Instead, use *shihan* to indicate that you are a Reiki teacher. The use of *sensei* may have been the source of Hawayo Takata referring to Usui Mikao, the founder of Reiki, as "Dr. Usui."

shashin chiryō hō (写真治療法): One of Usui's favorite healing methods, *shashin chiryō hō* means "photograph treatment method," and it is a long-distance method for administering Reiki. See also *enkaku chiryō hō*.

shihan (師範): This is the title used for teachers of Reiki in Japan. Translated as "instructor," *shihan* is the equivalent of Reiki Master or Reiki Master/Teacher in Western Reiki. See also *dai shihan* and *shihan-kaku*.

shihan-kaku (師範格): Meaning "assistant instructor," this title was historically given to *shinpiden* students who were permitted to teach only the *shoden* class. This was considered a trial period that prepared prospective students to teach others. The Jikiden Reiki Kenkyukai still uses this title today.

shingon (真言): *Shingon* is the Japanese term for *mantra,* literally "true word(s)." The names of the Reiki symbols in Western branches of Reiki are used as *shingon,* or mantras; this is not to be confused with *jumon,* which are written formulas comprised of kanji, whose power is released when spoken *and* drawn. *Shingon* may also refer to Shingon Shū (真言宗), a Buddhist sect that utilizes mantras and mudras.

shinpiden (神秘傳): *Shinpiden* is the third degree of Reiki, literally the "mystery teachings" in Japanese. After being initiated in the third degree, students may become *shihan* or Reiki teachers (Reiki Masters in the West). Many lineages now have broken down the third degree or level of Reiki into smaller, more accessible seminars, so that one is not required to become a teacher all at once.

shin shin kaizen (心身改善): Often rendered "mind and body improvement," "the expression *shin shin kaizen* occurs in the full name of Usui's Reiki system: Shin Shin Kaizen Usui Reiki Ryōhō, which means "Usui Reiki Healing Method for Improving the Heart-Mind and Body." An alternate translation, especially as it occurs in the *gokai,* is "improve your [heart-]mind and body: Usui Reiki Ryōhō." Note that *heart* (or *mind*) expressed as the *kokoro/shin* character, 心, precedes the word for *body;* Usui-sensei surely ordered them in this manner purposefully, thereby indicating that improving the mind allows the body to follow suit.

shinshūkyō (新宗教): *Shinshūkyō* literally means "new sect teachings." The *shinshūkyō* are also called Japanese New Religions or new religious movements (NRMs). They emerged in Japan beginning in the late nineteenth century. New spiritual practices flourished in Japan in the twentieth century, and they were often based upon older traditions, including Shinto, Buddhism, Hinduism, and Christianity. Reiki emerged during this period of rapid change and new spiritual movements; it's closely linked with several other similar movements that evolved contemporaneously. Most of them were treated with caution—sometimes even suppressed—by the Japanese government, but Usui Reiki Ryōhō enjoyed special treatment due to Usui's political and social connections and because of his reverence for the Meiji emperor.

Shintō (神道): Shinto is the native shamanic, animistic religious practice of Japan. Shinto had no formal name until Buddhism was brought to the nation in what was probably the sixth century C.E. Shinto is also called *kami no michi,* an alternate reading of the kanji. Its name is translated as "the way of the kami." Shinto has a strong reverence for nature and teaches a way of living in harmony unique to Japanese culture.

shirushi (印): Meaning "symbol," "sign," or "mark," this word is used to describe the Reiki symbols from the Japanese perspective. The symbols each have a specialized function, and they are introduced in *okuden* in most lineages of Reiki Ryōhō.

shizen jōka sayō (自然浄化作用): This term refers to a biological concept and translates as "natural purification action." *Shizen jōka sayō* is not unique to Reiki; it is a term widely used in allopathic and integrative medicine and in spiritual healing in Japan. In the context of Reiki Ryōhō, *shizen jōka sayō* is used to describe the body's normal accumulation and disposal of toxins, such as in discussing *byōsen*.

shoden (初傳 or 初伝): *Shoden* is the original name for the first degree of Reiki in Japanese. *Sho* (初) is "entrance," while *den* (傳) is "to transmit, convey." Together, it means "transmitting the entrance" or "entry-level teachings." This is the introduction to the system of Usui Reiki Ryōhō wherein the practitioner enters the stream of Reiki by direct transmission (the initiation or *reiju*) from his or her teacher.

tanden (丹田): Literally "red field," this term refers to centers of vital energy; it is pronounced *dantian* in Chinese. The most commonly referred to of the three centers is the lower *tanden* or *hara,* which is located two to three finger-widths below the navel. This is the "big motor" or "battery" that Takata referred to in her Reiki seminars, and it is the seat of both our life force and Reiki.

tanden chiryō (丹田治療): "*Tanden* treatment" is one of the original Japanese Reiki Techniques. See also *gedoku hō.*

teate (手当): *Teate* literally means "to apply the hands." Figuratively it means the laying on of hands for healing.

temizu (手水): *Temizu* is a specific form of purification used before entering Shinto temples and Buddhist shrines in Japan. Special basins and long-handled bamboo ladles are provided for visitors to cleanse themselves by washing their hands in a left-right-left pattern before also rinsing their mouths. This ceremony, including the pattern of left-right-left, has a familiar connection to *kenyoku hō* in Reiki Ryōhō.

Tennō (天皇): *Tennō* is the title of the Emperor of Japan, comprised of the kanji for "heaven" and "emperor," thus asserting that the imperial line is descended from the kami.

tenohira (手のひら or 掌): Meaning "palm," *tenohira* sometimes is used to indicate healing by the laying on of hands, such as in Reiki Ryōhō. See also *teate.*

tsūshin kōshū (通信講習): This term means "correspondence course."

Hawayo Takata received a correspondence course from the Hayashi Reiki Kenkyukai in Tokyo; the exact nature of these lessons has not been determined.

uchideshi (内弟子): *Uchideshi* means "inside student." An *uchideshi* is afforded additional access and inner, possibly secret, more advanced teachings by living with his or her teacher. This concept is special to Japanese culture; Hawayo Takata was Hayashi's *uchideshi*. This term is occasionally rendered as "apprentice" in English, although it does not convey the level of intimate, continuous support that *uchideshi* entails.

uchū ware soku, ware soku uchū (宇宙即我、即我宇宙): This phrase roughly means "you are (or I am) in the universe, and the universe is in you (me)." This is the core teaching that Usui-sensei transmitted after his experience of *anshin ritsumei*. Some of his students have interpreted it as "I exist in God, and God exists in me" and "I exist in enlightenment, and enlightenment exists in me." Takata is known to have shared this teaching with her early students in Hawaii.

Usui Reiki Ryōhō (臼井靈氣療法): *Usui Reiki Ryōhō* means "Usui spiritual energy healing method," which was translated as "Usui Method of Natural Healing" by Hawayo Takata and used on the certificates she issued. This is the name of the system of Reiki, which differentiates between it and the energy that *is* Reiki.

Usui Reiki Ryōhō Gakkai (臼井靈氣療法学会): *Gakkai* means "society," and thus this phrase represents the Usui Reiki Healing Method Society. The *gakkai* records its first president as being Usui-sensei himself, and it continues to practice in the way that it is believed he taught, as authentically as possible. Outsiders are not permitted access or entrance to the *gakkai,* although one seminal member, Doi Hiroshi, has made some *gakkai* teachings available through a branch of Reiki that he calls Gendai Reiki Hō (Modern Reiki Method). Gendai Reiki offers an approach that uses the best practices of both Eastern and Western lineages of Reiki.

Usui Shiki Ryōhō (臼井式療法): Usui-Style Healing Method is the system of Reiki as taught by Hawayo Takata; originally it was called

Usui Shiki Reiki Ryōhō (Usui-Style Reiki Healing Method). This serves as the origin of the Usui Method of Natural Healing that she referred to on her Reiki certificates. Western Lineages of Reiki may all be traced back to Usui Shiki Ryōhō.

wa (は): A particle used in the Japanese language to indicate the topic of a sentence or passage. It is used in the *gokai* to mark *kyō dake* ("today only") as the central theme of the five admonitions.

waka (和歌): *Waka* is a form of poetry consisting of a syllable count of 5-7-5-7-7. The Meiji emperor composed *waka* (called *gyosei* when written by an emperor), 125 of which were selected by Usui Mikao as teaching tools for the Usui Reiki Ryōhō Gakkai.

zui un (瑞雲): The *zui un* or "auspicious cloud" is a common motif in Asian art. Often depicted with a spiraling shape, the *zui un* represents the heavens (and therefore the home of the kami) and is also thought to bring good fortune. The spiral of the *zui un* motif is believed to have influenced the shape of the first *shirushi, choku rei.*

APPENDIX D

GLOSSARY OF NAMES

FOR MANY READERS, the cast of characters in the Reiki milieu may sound foreign, and many of the names do in fact sound similar. In light of this, I have compiled a list of people discussed throughout this book. Brief biographical information is provided below. Names are alphabetized according to the style in which they appear in the text. Thus, Japanese names are listed with the family name first, while Western names are listed with personal name first. Names of Japanese origin are provided in their original forms, with the hope that this will aid future researchers. The kanji provided are correct to the best of my knowledge, although many names have more than one spelling in Japanese.

Barbara Weber Ray (1941–?): Ray was one of Takata-sensei's twenty-two *shihan,* or Reiki Masters, and the first to defect from Takata's original teachings. Ray called her method Authentic Reiki, later changing the name to the Radiance Technique. She claimed to be the only Master who received the complete system of Reiki from Takata, alleging that there were actually seven levels rather than three. The Radiance Technique and its parent organization, the Radiance Technique International Association, still offer training in Ray's methods. Her current whereabouts and status are unknown. It was through one of Ray's students, Mitsui Mieko, that Western Reiki was transmitted to Japan after Takata's death.

Dave King (?–): Dave King is a Reiki teacher and author of *O-Sensei: A View of Mikao Usui*. King has made numerous spurious claims about Reiki history, many of which have been contradicted by subsequent research and publications by other members of the Reiki community. King teaches a revisionist style of Reiki called Usui Dō ("Way of Usui"), which he purports is a re-creation of Usui's original teachings prior to the founding of the Usui Reiki Ryōhō Gakkai.

Deguchi Onisaburō (出口　王仁三郎) (1871–1948): Born Ueda Kisaburō (上田　喜三郎), Deguchi Onisaburō is one of the founders and leaders of Shinto-derived Oomoto Kyō, one of the most prominent *shinshūkyō* to arise in Japan. Several ideas that are prominent in the original practices and principles of *dento Reiki* can also be found in Deguchi's teachings, as well as in traditional Shinto thought. Several Reiki researchers have suggested a connection between Oomoto Kyō and Usui Mikao, but there is no evidence to support these claims.

Doi Hiroshi (土居　裕) (1935–): Doi Hiroshi is a noted Reiki *shihan*, researcher, and (possibly former) member of the Usui Reiki Ryōhō Gakkai. He is best known for having founded the lineage known as Gendai Reiki Hō after his teacher, Koyama Kimiko, gave him permission to teach the *gakkai's* history and some of its techniques to outsiders. Doi first learned Western-style Reiki (the Radiance Technique) from a journalist, Mitsui Mieko, who was a student of Takata-trained Barbara Weber Ray. Doi has been one of the most important figures in bringing original practices and accurate history of *dento Reiki* to the world at large.

Eguchi Toshihiro (江口　俊博) (1873–1946): Eguchi was a student of Usui Mikao and a member of the Usui Reiki Ryōhō Gakkai. He maintained his membership in the *gakkai* for only two years before leaving to found his own healing system, Tenohira Ryōji. He was introduced to the *gakkai* by a woman named Tamura and therefore was not a personal friend of Usui-sensei prior to being admitted to the *gakkai,* as once thought by Reiki researchers. He cited the high class fees for Reiki training as his motive for leaving the *gakkai,* and his healing system was at one time very popular.

Frank Arjava Petter (1960–): Frank Arjava Petter (better known as Arjava or Arjava-sensei to his students) was born in Germany and at the age of eighteen moved to India to become a student of the spiritual teacher Osho. He would later study Reiki and become a teacher of Western Reiki. In the 1990s Arjava lived in Japan and was the first person to offer Reiki Master training in Western-style Reiki in Japan. He and his then-wife Chetna uncovered many important pieces of Reiki history, including Usui-sensei's memorial stone and publications used by the Usui Reiki Ryōhō Gakkai. Petter networked with several notable Japanese Reiki practitioners and *shihan,* including Ogawa Fumio, Oishi Tsutomu, and then-president of the Usui Reiki Ryōhō Gakkai, Koyama Kimiko. He travels extensively to teach Reiki and was the first person to offer Western audiences training in the original Japanese Reiki Techniques. Petter now serves as the vice chairperson of the Jikiden Reiki Kenkyukai and continues to research and teach Reiki. He is the author of ten books on Reiki Ryōhō.

Frans Stiene (1966–): Frans Stiene is a Reiki *shihan,* writer, and cofounder of the International House of Reiki. Stiene is the author of several books on Reiki, and his teachings and research emphasize the correlations between Japanese Buddhism and the philosophy of Usui Reiki Ryōhō.

Gōto Shinpei (後藤 新平) (1857–1929): Usui Mikao's former employer, Gōto was a much-beloved politician in Japan. He obtained a medical degree and worked in medicine and later in politics. He would eventually become the mayor of Tokyo, and during his term Usui would be invited to help the victims of the Great Kanto Earthquake (1923) with Reiki. It is through the political and military connections that Usui made during his tenure as Gōto's assistant that he was able to proliferate the practice of Usui Reiki Ryōhō.

Harry Kuboi (1930–2013): Kuboi was a resident of Hawaii and one of Takata's twenty-two *shihan.* He is the author of two books on Reiki, one of which consists of "channeled" information about the life of Usui and the origin of the system of Reiki. Kuboi also describes the concept of *byōsen* as he learned it from Hawayo Takata, although he does not write about it by name.

Hawayo Takata (高田 ハワヨ [Takada Hawayo*]) (1900–1980): Born Hawayo Hiromi Kawamura on the Big Island of Hawaii, Takata is best known for bringing Reiki out of Japan to the Western world. Takata called her style of Reiki practice Usui Shiki Ryōhō, meaning "Usui-Style Healing Method." A more complete biography of Takata is included in chapter 3.

Hayashi Chūjirō (林 忠次郎) (1880–1940): Hayashi-sensei enrolled in the Royal Naval Academy in 1899 and attained the rank of captain in the Japanese Navy. He oversaw logistics at harbors. He and his wife, Hayashi Chie, had two children. Around 1924 Hayashi met Usui Mikao and subsequently began to study Reiki Ryōhō. He became a *shihan* and opened a public Reiki clinic, purportedly because of his background in medicine. Hayashi left the Usui Reiki Ryōhō Gakkai on friendly terms to focus on his own association, the Hayashi Reiki Kenkyukai. Hayashi would go on to teach influential Reiki figures Hawayo Takata and Yamaguchi Chiyoko. Hayashi honorably took his own life in 1940 when pressured to supply the Japanese Navy with information about Hawaii, from where Hayashi had just returned after teaching Reiki. He left his wife, Chie, in charge of the Hayashi Reiki Kenkyukai. A more thorough discussion of Hayashi can be found in chapter 3.

Jojan Jonker (1956–): Jojan Jonker became a Reiki Master in 1998 and later went on to study interreligious spirituality at Radboud University in the Netherlands. Jonker completed his doctoral study on the transmigration of Reiki and published this as *Reiki: The Transmigration of a Japanese Spiritual Healing Practice.* Jonker is considered a *both-sider* in that he is

---

*The traditional romanization (and pronunciation) of 高田 is Takada in Japan; this is the pronunciation indicated in several articles in the *Hawaii Hochi*. Hawayo's husband's family probably immigrated to the Hawaiian Islands before the current standardized rules for transcribing Japanese words were put into practice, thereby resulting in the family name being recorded as Takata.

both an academic and a student of Reiki, and he is a member of the Reiki Alliance.

Justin Stein (?–): Justin Stein is a Reiki Master and academic (considered a *both-sider* like his colleague Jonker) who focuses on the history and development of Reiki. Stein has translated several Japanese articles about Reiki originally written in the 1930s, and he has published several academic papers about Reiki Ryōhō. Stein has access to the Takata Archives of the Reiki Alliance, and at the time of writing he has a forthcoming paper that will reveal new biographical details about Takata and her Reiki practice. In September 2017 Justin Stein finished his doctoral study on the topic of Takata and Reiki at Toronto University.

Kawakami Mataji (川上 又次) (?–?): A hands-on healing therapist who purportedly wrote and published a book about a different form of Reiki Ryōhō in 1914, Mr. Kawakami is thought to have practiced his own style of Reiki Ryōhō unrelated to that of Usui Mikao. Little else is known about him, and researchers are unsure whether copies of his book are extant today.

Kondō Masaki (近藤 正毅) (1933–2010): Mr. Kondō succeeded Mrs. Koyama as the seventh president of the Usui Reiki Ryōhō Gakkai. Kondō was apparently not interested in the spread of Reiki Ryōhō, and the Usui Reiki Ryōhō Gakkai's membership shrank under his leadership.

Koyama Kimiko (小山 君子) (1906–1999): Mrs. Koyama was the sixth president of the Usui Reiki Ryōhō Gakkai and the first female president, serving from 1975 to 1998. Koyama was Doi Hiroshi's teacher in the *gakkai,* and she assisted Frank Arjava Petter with his research in the 1990s. Koyama-sensei was considered a progressive leader in the *gakkai,* and under her stewardship the once-dwindling membership began to grow again.

Meiji Tennō (明治天皇) (1852–1912): Also called Meiji Taitei (明治大帝), meaning "Meiji, the Great." Emperor Meiji was one of the most influential figures in recent Japanese history. Under his rule political power was once again consolidated and returned to the imperial family. Meiji Tennō was responsible for the modernization and industrialization of Japan, and it is known that Usui Mikao looked up to him. Usui used Meiji's *gyosei* or *waka* poetry in his classes as tools to teach moral and spiritual lessons.

Mitsui Mieko (三井 ミエコ) (?–?): Ms. Mitsui was a journalist and resident of New York. She studied Reiki (as the Radiance Technique) under Barbara Weber Ray and initially brought this style of Reiki to Japan in 1985. Mitsui is credited as Doi Hiroshi's first Reiki teacher. She is often considered to be the first person to bring Western Reiki to Japan, even though Takata-sensei made at least one trip to Japan to teach Usui Shiki Ryōhō in the 1970s. During her time in Japan Mitsui discovered that Reiki Ryōhō had not died out in its home country as Takata had claimed earlier.

Nishina Masaki (仁科 まさき) (?–): Nishina is a Reiki researcher and teacher. He is a *dai shihan* (senior instructor) with the Jikiden Reiki Kenkyukai and a Reiki Master in Western-style Reiki. He is the author of *Reiki and Japan: A Cultural View of Western and Japanese Reiki.*

Ogawa Fumio (小川 二三男) (1906–1998): Ogawa-sensei originally learned *shinpiden* from his father, Ogawa Kozo (or Keizo), in 1943. Ogawa corresponded with Frank Arjava Petter (via one of Petter's Japanese students) and contributed techniques and historical anecdotes to Petter's research. Ogawa also wrote a booklet called "Everyone Can Do Reiki" that compiled his perspective of and lifelong experience with Reiki Ryōhō. This booklet has never been formally published; Ogawa freely gave copies of it to his students and other interested parties.

Phyllis Furumoto (1948–): Phyllis is Hawayo Takata's granddaughter and the current head of the Reiki Alliance, an organization dedicated to preserving Takata's teachings and style of Reiki. Phyllis learned Reiki from Takata at an early age and apprenticed with her as a Reiki *shihan* (Master) in the late 1970s just prior to Takata's death. In 1982 Phyllis gathered with many of the other *shihan* trained by Takata-sensei and they collectively formed the Reiki Alliance. The alliance recognizes Furumoto as the lineage-bearer and "grandmaster" of Usui Shiki Ryōhō (or Usui Shiki Reiki Ryōhō).

Robert N. Fueston (1975–): Robert Fueston is a Reiki teacher and author. He is a member of the Reiki Alliance and the founder of the Reiki Preservation Society, which aims to preserve the teachings and practices of Hawayo Takata. Fueston has researched Takata's Reiki thoroughly, personally studying with and interviewing many of her students. Fueston compiled much of his research into his first book, *The History and System of Usui Shiki Reiki Ryoho* volume 1 of *Reiki: Transmissions of Light*.

Sugano Wasaburō (菅野 和三郎) (?–?): Sugano Wasaburō was Yamaguchi Chiyoko's uncle; she lived with Sugano and his wife from the time she was in the third grade until adulthood. Sugano first studied Reiki Ryōhō with Hayashi Chūjirō in 1928 after the tragic loss of both of his children, and he was instrumental in founding the Daishōji branch of the Hayashi Reiki Kenkyukai in 1935. Mr. Sugano became a *shihan* in 1933, and he enrolled Chiyoko in the *shoden* and *okuden* seminar with Hayashi-sensei. Sugano taught Chiyoko how to perform *reiju* in the *shinpiden* seminar around 1940.

Suzuki Bizan (鈴木 美山) (?–?): Little is known of Dr. Suzuki, although a poem in his book *Kenzen no Genri* (Principles of Health) is the likeliest inspiration for Usui Mikao's *gokai*. Suzuki was a proponent of the New Thought Movement and may have been one of the early people propagating this ideology in Japan.

Takahashi Ichita (高橋 一太) (?–): Takahashi is the eighth and current president of the Usui Reiki Ryōhō Gakkai. Under his progressive leadership, the *gakkai* has begun to grow in membership again and is purportedly becoming more open to dialogue with other traditions of Reiki and with foreigners.

Taketomi Kan'ichi (武富 咸一) (1878–1960): Mr. Kan'ichi was the third president of the Usui Reiki Ryōhō Gakkai, and he began his term in 1935. The exact date that his term ended is unclear. Taketomi-sensei served in Japan's navy until 1941.

Tomita Kaiji (富田 魁二) (?–?): Tomita was a student of Usui Mikao in 1925 but left the Usui Reiki Ryōhō Gakkai to teach his own system of healing, Tomita-ryu Teate Ryōhō (Tomita Hands-on Healing Method). He published a book about Reiki in 1933, called *Reiki To Jinjutsu— Tomita-ryu Teate Ryōhō* (Reiki and the Art of Compassion: Tomita Hands-on Healing Method). Tomita's healing system has disappeared, as he left no successors.

Ueshiba Morihei (植芝 盛平) (1883–1969): The founder of the martial art aikido, Ueshiba was an adherent of Oomoto Kyō. He popularized the philosophy of *kotodama* through his teachings in aikido. Because Ueshiba and Usui lived in Japan at roughly the same time, there are a number of similarities in their respective teachings—both are rooted in the ideology of Japan itself and its spiritual traditions. Several Reiki researchers have made tenuous claims of a connection between Ueshiba and Usui, but there is no evidence that supports these statements.

Ushida Juzaburō (牛田 従三郎) (1865–1935): Mr. Ushida was the second president of the Usui Reiki Ryōhō Gakkai and is considered to be Usui Mikao's successor. Ushida served from 1926 until he died in 1935. Ushida was a rear admiral in the Japanese Navy, and he was a gifted calligrapher. Ushida brushed the most widely known copy of the *gokai,* and he also contributed his talent to the inscription of Usui's memorial stone in the Saihōji Temple cemetery.

Usui Mikao (臼井 甕男) (1865–1926): Founder of the system of Usui Reiki Ryōhō. Usui's lifelong quest for inner peace, or *anshin ritsumei,* fueled his accidental discovery and subsequent teaching of Usui Reiki Ryōhō. Usui was the first president of the *gakkai*; he served as president and taught Reiki from April 1922 until his death in March 1926. Usui Mikao taught over two thousand people his system of Reiki Ryōhō. A detailed account of his life and teachings is available in chapter 3.

Wanami Hōichi (和波 豊一) (1883–1975): Mr. Wanami served as the fifth president of the Usui Reiki Ryōhō Gakkai. The exact date that he began serving is unclear, but his term ended in 1975. Wanami-sensei also served in the Japanese Navy.

Watanabe Yoshiharu (渡辺 義治) (?–1960): Mr. Watanabe served as the fourth president of the Usui Reiki Ryōhō Gakkai; the dates of his term are unclear, but it is known that Watanabe-sensei led the *gakkai* after the war. Watanabe was a high school teacher, and he was the first civilian president of the *gakkai* (aside from Usui himself).

Yamaguchi Chiyoko (山口　千代子) (1921–2003): Born Iwamoto Chiyoko (presumably written 岩本　千代子), Chiyoko-sensei learned Reiki from Hayashi Chūjirō as a teenager in Daishōji, Ishikawa, in 1938. Chiyoko married Yamaguchi Shosuke in 1942, and the couple had four sons, including Tadao. In the late 1990s Mrs. Yamaguchi was encouraged to begin teaching Reiki Ryōhō as she learned it from Hayashi-sensei. With her son Tadao, she helped found the Jikiden Reiki Kenkyukai. More information on Yamaguchi Chiyoko can be found in chapter 3.

Yamaguchi Tadao (山口　忠夫) (1952–): Tadao is the son of Yamaguchi Chiyoko and the founder of the Jikiden Reiki Kenkyukai. He worked with his mother to collect evidence of Hayashi's teachings from their extended family who studied with Hayashi in the 1920s through the 1940s. Tadao-sensei is the current head of the Jikiden Reiki Kenkyukai and continues to engage in research for the betterment of the global Reiki community.

NOTES

CHAPTER 1. DEFINING REIKI

1. List summarized from Lübeck, Petter, and Rand, *Spirit of Reiki,* 53–60.
2. Lübeck, Petter, and Rand, *Spirit of Reiki,* 60.
3. International Center for Reiki Training, *Evidence Based History of Reiki,* 37.
4. Stiene, *Inner Heart of Reiki,* 15.
5. International Center for Reiki Training, *Evidence Based History of Reiki,* 36.
6. Doi, *Modern Reiki Method,* 32.
7. "Reiki Ryōhō Lecture Leaves a Big Impression," https://thescienceofsoul .wordpress.com/2014/04/19/19371127.

CHAPTER 2. LEARNING REIKI

1. Fueston, *Reiki: Transmissions of Light,* 209.
2. A more complete list can be found in Rand, *Reiki: The Healing Touch,* 144.
3. Petter, "Shoden and Okuden."
4. International Center for Reiki Training, *Evidence Based History of Reiki,* 24.
5. International Center for Reiki Training, *Evidence Based History of Reiki,* 98.
6. Fueston, *Reiki: Transmissions of Light,* 124.

CHAPTER 3. REIKI HISTORY

1. Jonker, *Reiki: The Transmigration,* 29.
2. Jonker, *Reiki: The Transmigration,* 170.
3. Jonker, *Reiki: The Transmigration,* 94.
4. Jonker, *Reiki: The Transmigration,* 174.
5. International Center for Reiki Training, *Evidence Based History of Reiki,* 41.
6. Jonker, *Reiki: The Transmigration,* 33.
7. Petter, *This Is Reiki,* 39.
8. Petter, *This Is Reiki,* 40.

9. Petter, *This Is Reiki*, 42.
10. Petter, "Shoden and Okuden."
11. Petter, *This Is Reiki*, 43.
12. Fueston, *Reiki: Transmissions of Light*, 22.
13. *Reiki Ryōhō no Shiori*, 43. Translation by author.
14. *Reiki Ryōhō no Shiori*, 43.
15. Jonker, *Reiki: The Transmigration*, 245.
16. Petter, *This Is Reiki*, 59.
17. International Center for Reiki Training, *Evidence Based History of Reiki*, 57.
18. International Center for Reiki Training, *Evidence Based History of Reiki*, 79.
19. International Center for Reiki Training, *Evidence Based History of Reiki*, 80.
20. Jonker, *Reiki: The Transmigration*, 220.
21. International Center for Reiki Training, *Evidence Based History of Reiki*, 43.
22. Fueston, *Reiki: Transmissions of Light*, 46.
23. Jonker, *Reiki: The Transmigration*, 253.
24. Fueston, *Reiki: Transmissions of Light*, 52.
25. Fueston, *Reiki: Transmissions of Light*, 52.
26. Fueston, *Reiki: Transmissions of Light*, 53.
27. Stein and Hirano in Fueston, *Reiki: Transmissions of Light*, 206–7. The original article from the *Hawaii Hochi* has been transcribed into modern Japanese and translated into English.
28. "Reiki Ryōhō's Hayashi Chūjirō Will Visit Hawaii." Reprinted online at http://jikiden-reiki-nishina.com/hawaii. Translation by author.
29. Fueston, *Reiki: Transmissions of Light*, 53.
30. Fueston, *Reiki: Transmissions of Light*, 57.
31. Fueston, *Reiki: Transmissions of Light*, 57.
32. Fueston, *Reiki: Transmissions of Light*, 58.
33. Nishina, *Reiki and Japan*, 130.
34. From Takata's Master certificate in International Center for Reiki Training, *Evidence Based History of Reiki*, 100.
35. U.S. National Archives and Records Administration, www.aetw.org/reiki_hayashi_travel_record.html.
36. Nishina, *Reiki and Japan*, 130.
37. Stein and Hirano in Jonker, *Reiki: The Transmigration*, 408.
38. Jonker, *Reiki: The Transmigration*, 367.
39. International Center for Reiki Training, *Evidence Based History of Reiki*, 70.
40. International Center for Reiki Training, *Evidence Based History of Reiki*, 71.
41. Yamaguchi, *Light on the Origins of Reiki*, 21.
42. Yamaguchi, *Light on the Origins of Reiki*, 30.

43. Yamaguchi, *Light on the Origins of Reiki*, 35.
44. Yamaguchi, *Light on the Origins of Reiki*, 50.
45. Inamoto and LaCore, *Shoden Manual*, 9.
46. Nishina, *Reiki and Japan*, 158.

CHAPTER 4. THE REIKI PRECEPTS

1. Stiene, www.ihreiki.com/blog/article/the_reiki_precepts_and_the_six_paramitas.
2. Deacon, "The Original Reiki Principles?" http://aetw.org/reiki_gokai_original.html.
3. Translation by Hyakuten Inamoto, as quoted in Rowland, *Reiki for the Heart and Soul*, 47.
4. Author's original translation.
5. Stiene, *Inner Heart of Reiki*, 61.
6. Author's original translation.
7. Mitchell, *Usui System of Natural Healing*.
8. Brown, *Living Reiki*, 52.
9. Lugenbeel, *Virginia Samdahl*, 75.
10. Twan, *Early Days of Reiki*, 14.
11. Stewart, *Reiki Touch*, 41–42.
12. Rowland, *Reiki for the Heart and Soul*, 36–37.
13. Horan, *Empowerment through Reiki*, 53.
14. International Center for Reiki Training, *Evidence Based History of Reiki*, 105.
15. Stiene, *Inner Heart of Reiki*, 59.
16. Henshall, *Guide to Remembering Japanese Characters*, 524.
17. Henshall, *Guide to Remembering Japanese Characters*, 71.
18. Henshall, *Guide to Remembering Japanese Characters*, 75.
19. Petter, *This Is Reiki*, 106.
20. Quoted from *Reiki Ryōhō Hikkei* in International Center for Reiki Training, *Evidence Based History of Reiki*, 34.
21. King, *O-sensei*, 47.
22. Stiene, *Inner Heart of Reiki*, 55.

CHAPTER 5. HOW REIKI HEALS

1. Lübeck, Petter, and Rand, *Spirit of Reiki*, 73.

CHAPTER 7. UNDERSTANDING *BYŌSEN*

1. Doi, *Modern Reiki Method for Healing*, 157.
2. Petter, *This Is Reiki*, 181.

3. Petter, *This Is Reiki,* 181.

4. Petter, *This Is Reiki,* 181.

5. List compiled from class notes, personal experience, and Petter, *This Is Reiki,* 192.

6. Petter, *This Is Reiki,* 180.

7. Haberly, *Reiki: Hawayo Takata's Story,* 58.

8. Kuboi, *All of Reiki,* 14.

9. Kuboi, *All of Reiki,* 17.

10. Kuboi, *All of Reiki,* 80.

11. Fulton and Prasad, *Animal Reiki,* 55–56.

CHAPTER 8. JAPANESE REIKI TECHNIQUES

1. Petter and Usui, *Original Reiki Handbook of Dr. Mikao Usui,* 15.

2. Fueston, *Reiki: Transmissions of Light,* 124.

3. From excerpt of Takata's diary as quoted in Petter, *This Is Reiki,* 227.

4. Author's original translation.

5. Doi, *Modern Reiki Method for Healing,* 125.

6. Doi, *Modern Reiki Method for Healing,* 125.

7. Rand, *Reiki: The Healing Touch,* 56.

8. Petter, *This Is Reiki,* 241.

9. Doi, *Modern Reiki Method for Healing,* 159.

10. Petter, *This Is Reiki,* 246.

CHAPTER 9. PRACTICING REIKI

1. International Center for Reiki Training, *Evidence Based History of Reiki,* 35.

CHAPTER 12. ADDITIONAL REIKI TECHNIQUES

1. Beckett, *Reiki: The True Story,* 69–70.

2. Fueston, *Reiki: Transmissions of Light,* 89–90.

3. Gray and Gray, *Hand to Hand,* 108.

4. Gray and Gray, *Hand to Hand,* 148.

5. Fueston, *Reiki: Transmissions of Light,* 128.

CHAPTER 15. THE FIRST SYMBOL: *CHOKU REI*

1. Jonker, *Reiki: The Transmigration,* 409.

2. Yamaguchi, *Light on the Origins of Reiki,* 147.

3. Nishina, *Reiki and Japan,* 145.

4. Lübeck and Hosak, *Big Book of Reiki Symbols,* 421.

5. Lübeck and Hosak, *Big Book of Reiki Symbols,* 421.

6. Takata to Doris Duke, December 19, 1978.
7. Takata to Doris Duke, December 19, 1978.
8. Doi, *Modern Reiki Method for Healing*, 62.
9. Gleason, *Spiritual Foundations of Aikido*, as quoted in Stiene, *Inner Heart of Reiki*, 65.
10. Nishina, *Reiki and Japan*, 145.

CHAPTER 16. THE SECOND SYMBOL: *SEI HEKI*

1. Petter, *This Is Reiki*, 153.
2. Stevens, *Sacred Calligraphy of the East*, 2.
3. Stevens, *Sacred Calligraphy of the East*, 4.
4. Stevens, *Sacred Calligraphy of the East*, 25.
5. Stevens, *Sacred Calligraphy of the East*, 26.
6. Doi, *Modern Reiki Method for Healing*, 66.
7. Jonker, *Reiki: The Transmigration*, 300.
8. Petter, *This Is Reiki*, 158.
9. Petter, *This Is Reiki*, 158.
10. Strübin, *L'essence*, 25–26.
11. Lübeck and Hosak, *Big Book of Reiki Symbols*, 168.
12. Yamaguchi, *Light on the Origins of Reiki*, 150.
13. Jonker, *Reiki: The Transmigration*, 409.
14. Yamaguchi, *Light on the Origins of Reiki*, 150.
15. Inamoto and LaCore, *Chuden Manual*, 8.
16. Lübeck and Petter, *Reiki Best Practices*, 116–20.

CHAPTER 17. THE THIRD SYMBOL: *HON SHA ZE SHŌ NEN*

1. Lübeck and Hosak, *Big Book of Reiki Symbols*, 334.
2. Lübeck and Hosak, *Big Book of Reiki Symbols*, 335.
3. Doi, *Modern Reiki Method for Healing*, 66.
4. An interview with Doi Hiroshi, founder of Gendai Reiki, in International Center for Reiki Training, *Evidence Based History of Reiki*, 57.
5. Stiene, *Inner Heart of Reiki*, 77.
6. Stiene, *Inner Heart of Reiki*, 77.
7. Phyllis Furumoto as quoted in Jonker, *Reiki: The Transmigration*, 303. Note that this is a poetic rather than literal translation of the kanji.
8. Stiene, *Inner Heart of Reiki*, 78.
9. Lübeck and Hosak, *Big Book of Reiki Symbols*, 341.
10. Lübeck and Hosak, *Big Book of Reiki Symbols*, 347.

11. Williams, *Chinese Symbolism and Art Motifs*, 86.
12. Lübeck and Hosak, *Big Book of Reiki Symbols*, 344.
13. Lübeck and Hosak, *Big Book of Reiki Symbols*, 345.
14. Lübeck and Hosak, *Big Book of Reiki Symbols*, 345.
15. Rowland, *Complete Book of Traditional Reiki*, 18.

CHAPTER 18. MORE JAPANESE REIKI TECHNIQUES

1. Petter, *This Is Reiki*, 242.
2. Petter, *This Is Reiki*, 243.
3. Stiene, *Inner Heart of Reiki*, 148.
4. Doi, *Modern Reiki Method for Healing*, 160.
5. Doi, *Modern Reiki Method for Healing*, 160.
6. Lübeck and Hosak, *Big Book of Reiki Symbols*, 329.
7. Yamaguchi, *Light on the Origins of Reiki*, 150–51.
8. Yamaguchi, *Light on the Origins of Reiki*, 150.
9. Lübeck and Hosak, *Big Book of Reiki Symbols*, 329.
10. Yamaguchi, *Light on the Origins of Reiki*, 151.
11. Petter, *This Is Reiki*, 234.
12. Petter, *This Is Reiki*, 235.

CHAPTER 19. ADDITIONAL *OKUDEN* TOOLS AND TECHNIQUES

1. Thakore and Thakore, *21 Power Tools of Reiki*, 123.

BIBLIOGRAPHY

Beckett, Don. *Reiki: The True Story*. Berkeley, Calif.: Frog Books, 2009.

Brown, Fran. *Living Reiki: Takata's Teachings*. Mendocino, Calif.: LifeRhythm, 1992.

Deacon, James. "The Original Reiki Principles?" http://aetw.org/reiki_gokai _original.html.

Doi Hiroshi. *A Modern Reiki Method for Healing*. Revised ed. Southfield, Mich.: International Center for Reiki Training, 2014.

Fueston, Robert N. *Reiki: Transmissions of Light*. Vol. 1, *The History and System of Usui Shiki Reiki Ryoho*. N.p.: self-published, 2016.

Fulton, Elizabeth, and Kathleen Prasad. *Animal Reiki: Using Energy to Heal the Animals in Your Life*. Berkeley, Calif.: Ulysses Press, 2006.

Gleason, William. *Aikido and Words of Power: The Sacred Sounds of Kototama*. Rochester, Vt.: Destiny Books, 2009.

Gray, John Harvey, and Lourdes Gray. *Hand to Hand: The Longest-Practicing Reiki Master Tells His Story*. N.p.: Xlibris Corporation, 2002.

Haberly, Helen. *Reiki: Hawayo Takata's Story*. Olney, Md.: Archedigm, 1990.

Henshall, Kenneth G. *A Guide to Remembering Japanese Characters*. North Clarendon, Vt.: Tuttle Publishing, 1998.

Horan, Paula. *Empowerment through Reiki*. Twin Lakes, Wisc.: Lotus Press, 1998.

Inamoto Hyakuten and Cerise LaCore. *Kōmyō Reiki Kai Shoden (First Degree) Manual*. N.p.: Kōmyō Reiki Kai International Association, 2014.

———. *Kōmyō Reiki Kai Chuden (Second Degree) Manual*. N.p.: Kōmyō Reiki Kai International Association, 2014.

———. *Kōmyō Reiki Kai Okuden (Third Degree) Manual*. N.p.: Kōmyō Reiki Kai International Association, 2014.

International Center for Reiki Training. *An Evidence Based History of Reiki*. Southfield, Mich.: International Center for Reiki Training, 2015.

Jonker, Jojan. *Reiki: The Transmigration of a Japanese Spiritual Healing Practice.* Zürich: Lit Verlag, 2016.

King, Dave. *O-sensei: A View of Mikao Usui.* Second ed. N.p.: 2006.

Kuboi, Harry. *All of Reiki: Book II.* Honolulu, Hawaii: Hawaii Reiki Center, 1996.

Leland, Kurt. *Rainbow Body: A History of the Western Chakra System from Blavatsky to Brennan.* Lake Worth, Fla.: Ibis Press, 2016.

Lübeck, Walter, and Mark Hosak. *The Big Book of Reiki Symbols.* Translated by Christine M. Grimm. Twin Lakes, Wisc.: Lotus Press, 2006.

Lübeck, Walter, and Frank Arjava Petter. *Reiki Best Practices: Wonderful Tools of Healing for the First, Second, and Third Degree of Reiki.* Twin Lakes, Wisc.: Lotus Press, 2003.

Lübeck, Walter, Frank Arjava Petter, and William Lee Rand. *The Spirit of Reiki: The Complete Handbook of the Reiki System.* Translated by Christine M. Grimm. Twin Lakes, Wisc.: Lotus Press, 2001.

Lugenbeel, Barbara D. *Virginia Samdahl: Reiki Master Healer.* Norfolk, Va.: Grundwald and Radcliff Publishers, 1984.

Maestro Myoren. *Seimei Reiki Ryoho: Un Manual de Reiki Shinto.* N.p.: Seimei Publishing, 2016.

Mitchell, Paul David. *The Usui System of Natural Healing.* Revised ed. Coeur d'Alene, Idaho: The Reiki Alliance, 1985.

Mochizuki Toshitaka and Kaneko Miyuki. *Chō Kantan Iyashi no Te.* Tokyo, Japan: Tama Publishing Co., Ltd., 2003.

Nishina, Masaki. "Hayashi's Activities in Hawaii." Jikiden Reiki by Masaki Nishina. http://jikiden-reiki-nishina.com/hawaii. Accessed July 26, 2017.

———. 日本と靈氣、そしてレイキ *(Japan and [Traditional] Reiki and [Western] Reiki).* N.p.: self-published, 2014.

———. *Reiki and Japan: A Cultural View of Western and Japanese Reiki.* Edited by Amanda Jayne. N.p.: self-published, 2017.

Petter, Frank Arjava. "Shoden and Okuden" (seminar, Jikiden Reiki Kenkyukai, Orlando, Fla., May 2016).

———. *This Is Reiki.* Twin Lakes, Wisc.: Lotus Press, 2012.

Petter, Frank Arjava, Tadao Yamaguchi, and Chujiro Hayashi. *The Hayashi Reiki Manual.* Twin Lakes, Wisc.: Lotus Press, 2003.

Petter, Frank Arjava, and Usui Mikao. *The Original Reiki Handbook of Dr. Mikao Usui.* Twin Lakes, Wisc.: Lotus Press, 2003.

Rand, William Lee. *Reiki: The Healing Touch.* Revised ed. Southfield, Mich.: International Center for Reiki Training, 2011.

"Reiki Ryōhō's Hayashi Chūjirō Will Visit Hawaii." *Hawaii Hochi,*

September 30, 1937, p. 7. Reprinted online at http://jikiden-reiki-nishina.com/hawaii.

"Reiki Ryōhō Lecture Leaves a Big Impression—A Great Success with Over 200 Attending." *Hawaii Hochi,* November 27, 1937, p. 4. Reprinted online at http://jikiden-reiki-nishina.com/hawaii and https://thescienceofthesoul.wordpress.com/2014/04/19/19371127.

Reiki Ryōhō no Shiori [靈氣療法のしおり]. Kazuwa Toyokazu, ed. Tokyo, Japan: Usui Reiki Ryoho Gakkai, 1974.

Rowland, Amy Z. *The Complete Book of Traditional Reiki: Practical Methods for Personal and Planetary Healing.* Rochester, Vt.: Healing Arts Press, 2010.

———. *Reiki for the Heart and Soul: The Reiki Principles as Spiritual Pathwork.* Rochester, Vt.: Healing Arts Press, 2008.

Stevens, John. *Sacred Calligraphy of the East.* Third ed. Boston: Shambhala Publications, Inc., 1995.

Stewart, Judy-Carol. *Reiki Touch: The Essential Handbook.* Second ed. Houston, Tex.: The Reiki Touch, Inc., 1995.

Stiene, Frans. *The Inner Heart of Reiki.* Winchester, U.K.: Ayni Books, 2015.

———. "The Reiki Precepts and the Six Paramitas." www.ihreiki.com/blog/article/the_reiki_precepts_and_the_six_paramitas.

Stiene, Frans, and Bronwen Steine. *The Japanese Art of Reiki.* New York: O Books, 2005.

———. *The Reiki Sourcebook.* New York: O Books, 2003.

Strübin, Barbara Chinta. *L'essence Cristalline du Reiki.* Romont, Switzerland: Recto Verseau, 2005.

Takata, Hawayo K., to Doris Duke, December 19, 1978. Doris Duke Papers, Doris Duke Charitable Foundation Historical Archives, David M. Rubenstein Rare Book & Manuscript Library, Duke University.

Thakore, Abhishek, and Usha Thakore. *21 Power Tools of Reiki: A Guide to Maximise the Power of Reiki.* New Delhi: Pustak Mahal, 2010.

Twan, Anneli, ed. *Early Days of Reiki: Memories of Hawayo Takata.* Hope, B.C.: Morning Star Productions, 2005.

U.S. National Archives and Records Administration. Manifest of *M.S. 'Chichibu Maru.'* Reprinted at www.aetw.org/reiki_hayashi_travel_record.html. Accessed July 26, 2017.

Williams, C. A. S. *Chinese Symbolism and Art Motifs.* North Clarendon, Vt.: Tuttle Publishing, 2006. First published in Shanghai in 1914.

Yamaguchi, Tadao. *Light on the Origins of Reiki.* Translated by Ikuko Hirota. Twin Lakes, Wisc.: Lotus Press, 2007.

INDEX